#1 Unconditional LOVE

A Mother Remembers
Her Bipolar Son

CAROL L. NIEMANN

Table of Content

INTRODUCTION

On January 14, 2006, I lost my son Timothy. He was forty-two years old. He stole a car and was in a horrific one car accident, and died four days later. He had been diagnosed with bipolar disorder when he was twenty-nine.

Bipolar disorder, sometimes called manic-depressive disorder, causes mood swings that range from the lows of depression to highs of mania. Some people experience mood shifts only a few times a year, others as often as several a day. It varies from person to person. Some are bothered more by the depression, others by the manic state. Timothy was diagnosed as a rapid cycler, meaning that he would have four or more mood shifts in a year. Bipolar disorder seems to run in families. A person with bipolar disorder suffers horribly, and anyone who loves them does too.

To look at Tim, you would think he was the perfect son. Good looking and well built, he had a big smile, dressed well, and liked people, especially small children and the elderly. He had a good sense of humor. He was fun to be with when his disorder was under control. Anything I didn't understand, he could explain to me.

I knew he suffered with the disorder, but I didn't know to what extent until he passed away and I went through his files. It was quite an eye opener. His life was chaos, but his files were in perfect order.

I loved Timothy so deeply and tried so hard to help him. After his death, many of his old friends told me that they are where they are today because of Tim. My father always taught me that there is a reason for everything, and while sometimes we can't see it, we just have to believe that God has one. It took me months after Tim's death to come up with reasons. Here are a few:

1. Tim made me stronger.

2. His journal and the papers from his file are Being used in the Polk County Sheriff's Crisis Intervention Classes in helping the deputies better understand the mentally ill.

3. People come to me to talk about a family member who is suffering with the disorder, and I try to help by listening.

4. I know Tim doesn't have to suffer anymore, and I know he is happy that his words are helping people.

I loved him dearly, but I would get very angry with him too, for the things he did. Maybe angry isn't the right word - hurt and sad are more accurate words. I hope this story will help people have a better understanding of their family member who is suffering with bipolar disorder.

**Welcome to My Life
And My Son's!**

1

My Life

When I was growing up in the 1930s and 40s, life was very different from today. My father was the most important person in our family, as in most families. At the dinner table the food was passed to him first, for Mother had told us that Dad worked hard to give us what we had. My two sisters and I were to be quiet and act like young ladies. Dad threatened that he would take us downstairs to the coal bin and spank us, but that never happened, although my sisters like to say, I was the only one who made it to the first step. Dad was so much fun. Mother was more serious and usually would be, either in the kitchen, cooking and cleaning, or upstairs, sewing. I remember Mother spanking one of my sisters, for lying to her. I knew I wasn't going to lie, because I didn't want to get a spanking. In grade school, the teachers used to take bad boys out into the hall and shut the door and then you would hear the whoop of a wooden paddle on their backsides, and oh, did those poor boys holler. To this day, I can still hear it.

One time my sister and I were throwing a tennis ball back and forth to each other in the living room, and my Mother in the kitchen, heard her collection of tea cups rattle. She hollered to Dad, "Arthur, talk to those girls." His response "girls how are you?" We, of course, stopped throwing the tennis ball and started laughing. But poor Mother, all we heard out of the kitchen was a loud "Arrrthurrr." Mother at one time had a dressmaker's shop on the better side of town, but after a year or so she gave it up. The landlord drank a great deal and it embarrassed her, when he came in drunk. Mother didn't drive, so Dad had to take her and pick her up, and eventually it all became too much for her. Many of her customers started coming to our house instead. She made many wedding dresses, for neighbors, girls from church, and of course, my sisters and me. In fact, she made not only our wedding dresses but all of our attendants, as well as her own.

My Dad had a great love of nature, gardening, people, and most importantly a love of God. My Mother was a fantastic seamstress and was very artistic. I don't remember Dad ever missing church on Sunday. Of course, I would be right behind him. He didn't go too many places without me tagging along. Mother once told me, after I had a family of my own, that she had learned many things from Dad. One of the most important was how a family should be. In her youth, Mother's life had not been especially happy. Dad always seemed to be happy, and he would talk and laugh with people whether he knew them or not. I loved being with him.

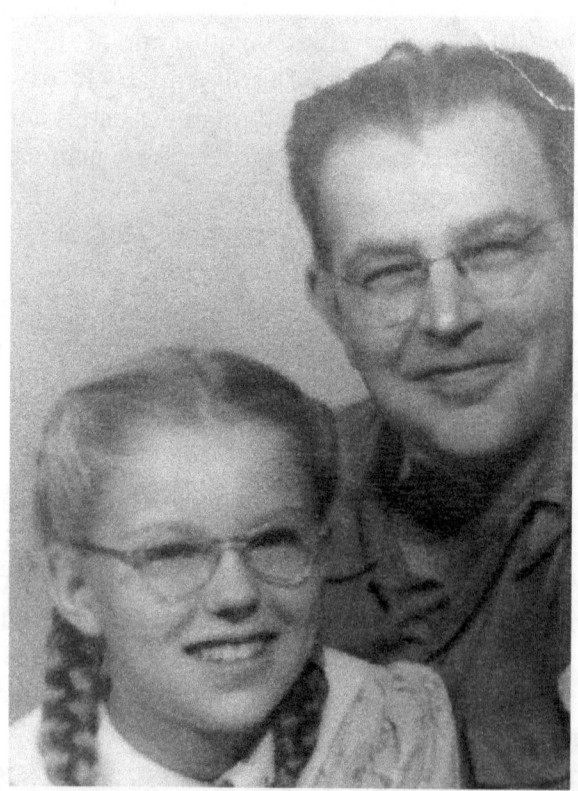

Carol and Arthur (her father)

I attended a small Lutheran grade school, in a two room school house, then off to a public high school. We didn't have a lot of money, but our parents always saw to it that we had what we really needed. Since my mother was such a great seamstress, we girls always had nice looking clothes. Having only girls in the family we could share the clothes, but you do know who received all the hand me downs.

We were a close family, even with being such a big difference in our ages. Betty was born first, ten years later Mary Ann, and four years after that, I came along. Dad worked in a factory from three o'clock in the afternoon till midnight. The weekends were when we could do things as a family. Even when I was in high school, if friends called to see if I wanted to do something with them, I always asked my parents what the family was planning to do. If we were even just going for a car ride somewhere, I would tell my friends I couldn't go with them. Sometimes the ride would be to a state park or to a river for a picnic lunch. We liked being together, and Dad always made it fun.

When I was trying to decide what I wanted to do as a career, law enforcement was very high on my list. My godfather was an Indiana state policeman and my favorite uncle was a city policeman. My mother and older sister said that law enforcement would be a terrible career; it would be depressing, and I would be around criminals most of the time. So I decided during my high school years that I wanted to be a teacher. I attended Indiana Central College, a small school in Indianapolis. My best friend Bernice, from high school also went there. We looked somewhat alike. We were about the same height, blond hair, and glasses and many people thought we were twins. One day she asked if I had a date yet for a dance that was coming up, and I did not. She said a friend of her boyfriend was interested in me, and she fixed me up with a blind date for the dance. Paul, the blind date, and I hit it off very well, and by the middle of my second year in College, we had decided to get married the following June, when Paul graduated from Butler University. I sometimes regret that I didn't finish school, for I loved children and also the teaching, but I also feel God had a reason: it gave me a lot of time for our own children.

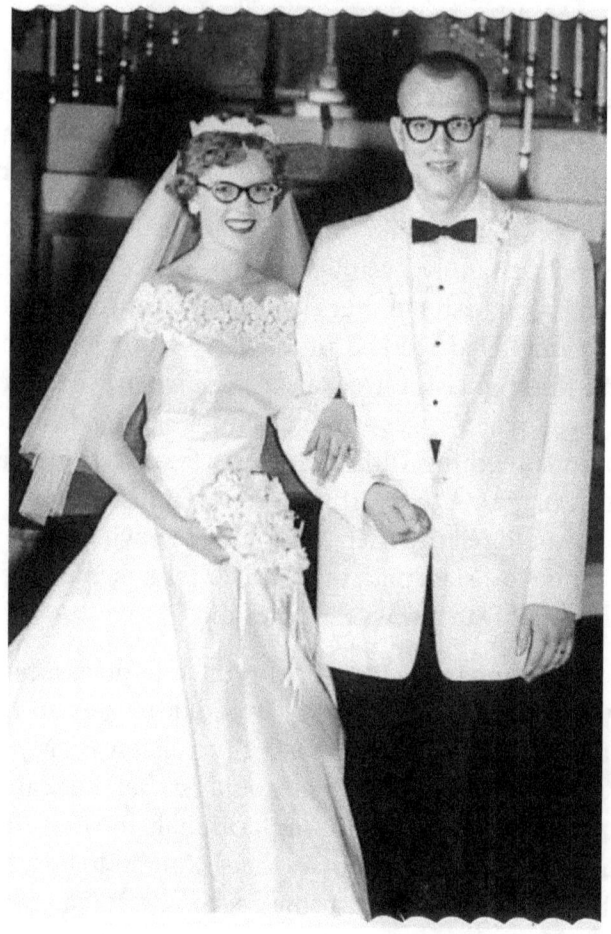

Carol and Paul (6-15-57)

On the day we were married, Paul received his Army reserve papers to report for active duty in two weeks, for a six month tour. So I lived with my parents, and Paul went off to Fort Leonard Wood, Missouri. When he came back, we found an apartment, and by then I was very pregnant. In April of 1958, we had a baby girl. She was born on Easter Sunday. Oh, we were so thrilled. By the time she was six months old; she had blond curly hair and was adorable. Paul was data processing manager of a grocery chain, and in October he was transferred to Memphis, Tennessee. It was hard to leave our families, but we were excited about a new adventure.

Memphis was so different from Indianapolis. The big Mississippi River, the antebellum homes, the cotton fields, and the different way of life. Segregation was big then in the South. Oh, so many rules. When we went to get our new driver's license, we found that black people could not enter by the same door as we did. Of course, there were the notorious black and white drinking fountains. I thought that was terrible, but the thing that really upset me was that black children were only allowed to go to the Memphis Zoo on Thursday afternoon. I thought that was horrible.

We lived in an apartment complex. Our neighbors were terrific. We would get together in the evenings for cards or a potluck dinner. They raved about Beth Anne. They said she looked like a little china doll. She was always so neat and clean.

One day, a neighbor knocked on our back door and she had a little girl by the hand, covered in dirt from head to toe. The woman was laughing, and said, "I think this is your little girl, but I'm not sure." Well, it was Beth Anne. The little boys had been throwing dirt up in the air and I think most of it had landed on her. Her eyelids were caked with it. She had a nice long, bubble bath, and was a little china doll once again. Beth Anne was a very quiet, sweet little girl. I cannot remember her ever throwing a temper tantrum. One Sunday in Church, we put Beth Anne in the nursery and she looked a little sad. We stayed outside the nursery door to see if she was going to get too upset to be left, but she seemed to get interested in the other children, so we went into the Church. Just as the organ music started, we noticed the Pastor leave the altar for a few minutes. We thought he must have forgotten something. After Church, when we went to get Beth from the nursery, the ladies told us, "Pastor heard Beth Anne cry and he came in and held her and talked to her. She settled down and has been very good." We could not believe he would do that, and we thanked him. He said she was a special little girl.

Mother flew down to Memphis in February of 1960, because I was about to give birth for a second time. The baby wasn't cooperating, and it was a week past the due date. Mother wrote a letter to Dad, stating that she could use a little money, she was running low. In those days people didn't call long distance unless it was an emergency. In a few days, Mother received a letter from Dad with a quarter in it. "Oh, that man!" she said. The next day, along came another letter from Dad with some money for Mom. Dad never changed, and everyone loved him. He could drive Mother crazy at times, for he loved teasing her. Finally Susan Kay arrived on February 17. When we brought the baby home from the hospital, I called the pediatrician and told him that she had little white bumps on her abdomen. He asked a few questions and told me to get a piece of paper and a pencil - not just a scrap of paper, but a tablet. He said it was very important to do exactly as he told me. First, bathe the baby every morning with Phisoderm cleanser. Secondly, sterilize a needle and open the bumps and immediately place a pad of cotton, which has been soaked in alcohol, on her belly for ten minutes. After that, you may dress her. Of course, she screamed when the alcohol was placed on her, and I would pick her up and love her and sing to her with tears running down my face too. It wasn't until she was healed that he told me, the bumps were a staphylococcus infection, that if it had not been caught when it was, it could have been tragic.

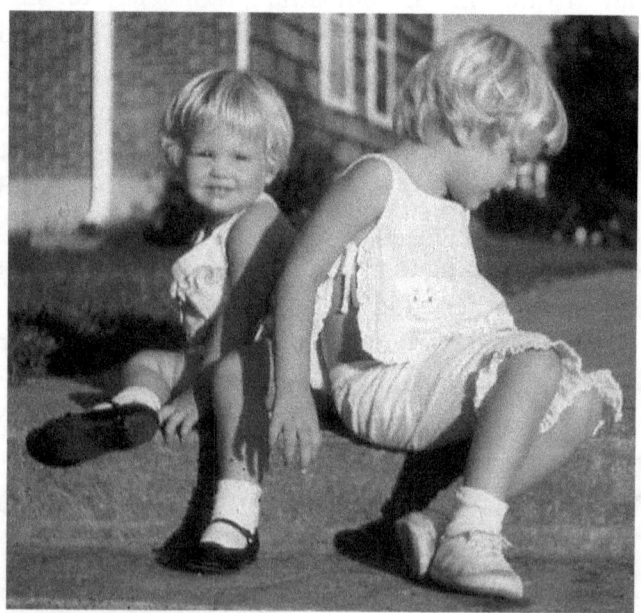

Susan Kay and Beth Anne

When Susan was able to sit up, the girls started entertaining each other. We enjoyed taking them to the zoo and playing along the river. Our weekends were devoted to having fun as a family. When possible, my parents would come down to visit and oh, how they enjoyed seeing the two little blonds. Susan was our little Dutch girl, with a round face and a ready smile. My mother always said if you had a hundred children, they would all look and act differently. Our two girls were very different from each other. By then, Mother and Dad had six grandchildren. Dad said some of the men at work couldn't believe he would waste his vacation going to see his kids and his grandkids. He told them he loved them and thoroughly enjoyed being around them.

On our way to church on Sundays, we would pass Graceland, Elvis's home. Those were the days when Elvis Presley was going strong. We never were able to see him; he would get mobbed if he went out in public. In the wee hours of the morning he would rent places, such as the amusement park, for himself and his friends. That was the only way he could do things.

We had just gotten comfortable in Memphis when Paul was transferred again. Halfway through 1961 we took up residence in Sioux City, Iowa. That was a different way of life, too. At that time it looked like a scene from 'Gunsmoke.' I expected to see Matt Dillon riding over the hill at any time. One day I took both girls into town with me to look for curtains for our new home. Downtown Sioux City was very small compared to Indianapolis and Memphis. Beth Anne always stayed right with me, but Susan was an explorer. All of a sudden, Susan was gone. I told the clerk right away that my little girl was missing, and she notified the other clerks. Soon we all were calling Susan and looking everywhere. Then two women walked into the store and said to a clerk, "Did you know a little girl is sitting on the couch in the window?" One of the women thought Susan was a manikin, but the other one said "She is real." She waved to Susan, who of course, waved right back. Needless to say, I tried not to shop with both girls by myself again

In the summer of 1962, my parents and my sister Mary Ann, her husband and their three children drove out to Sioux City, and we all took off for Yellowstone National Park. We've talked about it since and we don't know how we managed it. There were six adults, five small children, food for a week, luggage, potty chair, items to keep the kids amused, and, of course, cameras, - and all of this was in two cars, not vans. Believe it or not, we saw everything there was to see and enjoyed every minute of it. None of us had ever been West, so it was all new and exciting. We stayed in motels and cooked our food in parks. On our trip we saw the Badlands, Wall Drug store, the Black Hills, Mount Rushmore, Custer State Park, Wind Cave National Park, Yellowstone National Park, and Teton National Park. We saw bears, moose, elk, big horn sheep, mountain goats, prairie dogs, donkeys, and things I have probably forgotten. At every turn, we would explain, "Oh, look at that," and the cameras would click. It was the highlight of all of our trips, a lot of family fellowship and just plain fun. We have been West in recent years and it made us very glad we went in 1962 when the roads weren't so crowded and the West looked like it should, without all the casinos, and parking garages.

2

Tim's Early Years

In the fall of 1963, we had just found out we would be having another baby in the spring, when Paul received word we would be transferred back to our hometown of Indianapolis. Everyone was delighted. My parents said we could move in with them, till we got our own place. We had always rented homes during our stays in other cities, but now we bought a lot and found a builder to build our first home.

I was the youngest grandchild and was born on my paternal grandfather's birthday, October 3rd, and our new baby, was the youngest grandchild, was due to be born on his maternal grandfather's birthday. My dad's birthday was May 7 and I went into the hospital to deliver our new baby on that day, but Timothy Brandt Niemann was born a little after midnight, so he was a May 8 baby. He weighed in at a whopping nine pounds fifteen and one half ounces. I awoke to the nurse asking the doctor why he didn't put his thumb on the scale and make it an even ten pounds. Whenever the nurse brought baby Tim from the nursery to my hospital room, she would carry him and sing to him all the way. I always knew when he was coming, by the singing.

Tim was a good baby, thank goodness, so we didn't keep my parents up at night. When he was a few months old, we were able to move into our new four bedroom home in Wanamaker, a suburb of Indianapolis. It was close to a Lutheran school and church. One of my sisters, Mary Ann, lived in the area; her family were members of the church too, and their children went to the school there. It was so nice to be close to our families and be together for holidays and birthdays once again. Beth Anne was starting first grade that year. The next year, Susan started kindergarten. So then it was Tim and I at home. It was nice living so close to Mary Ann, for we could take turns looking after each other's children. There were three girls and a boy in their family and her youngest was a month older than Tim, so they would start to school together. Betty and her family lived in New Palestine, a little further out of Indianapolis. They had two girls and a boy. Our children all basically were about the same age. Their children went to a different Lutheran school, and our children often competed against each other in basketball and track.

Tim's and Dad's birthdays being a day apart didn't stop them from celebrating their birthdays by going out for dinner, just the two of them. I remember the first time Dad took him out to a buffet. Tim must have been five years old then, and the waitress asked Dad if it would be one adult's and one child's plate. Dad of course said yes, but when the waitress handed Tim a plate with a chicken leg on it, Dad saw Tim's face and quickly said, let's make it two adults. Tim was much happier, for he was a good eater. He didn't care for sweets as the girls did.

The girls soon learned in order to keep their little brother out of their bedrooms, they had to hang creepy crawlers on the door knobs. He did not like bugs. By the time Tim was in kindergarten, it was already obvious that he was very intelligent. People would say to him, "You are really going to be something when you grow up". Years later, he told me that statement bothered him. He always wondered what he was supposed to be. He and his cousin Kristine would discuss topics that were over the heads of their classmates. Tim knew that I had not attended kindergarten. One day when he asked me a question about something he had learned in school, he was amazed that I would know the answer, because I hadn't been to kindergarten.

It didn't take the two cousins long to figure out that Santa wasn't real. They saw too many Santas and they all looked different. Tim's kindergarten teacher sent home a note: PLEASE TELL TIM NOT TO TELL THE OTHER KIDS THERE ISN'T A SANTA CLAUS! Mary Ann's son Johnny gave Tim a nickname: "Webster, the walking, talking dictionary". The name stuck with him for a long time.

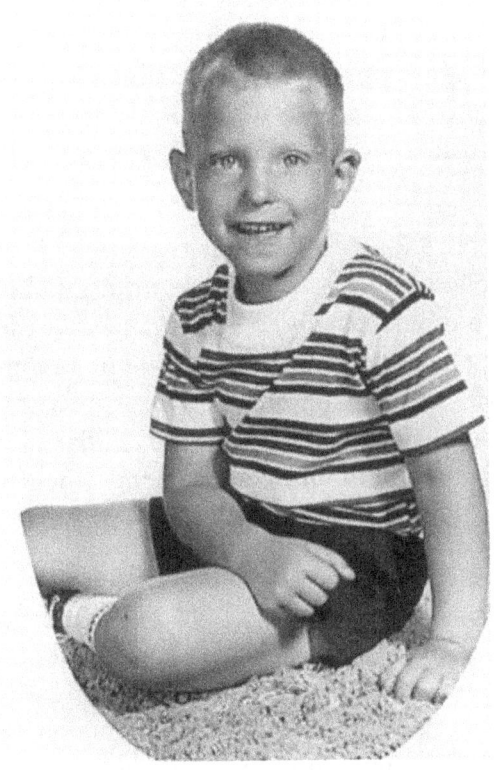

Timothy

One peculiar habit Tim had as a child, he was thumping his head on his pillow to get to sleep. It became annoying to us when we would go camping. We had a pop- up camper, and when he thumped his head, the whole trailer rocked. He slept on the bed below Paul's and mine, and I would hold his head down till he was sound asleep. That way I didn't have to hear the girls fussing about him.

All of our vacations were camping trips. We all loved the outdoors, except that when we had to use outdoor toilets, Beth Anne could sure complain. None of us enjoyed them, but Beth was the big objector. When we would go out West, the national forests did not have many facilities, but oh, did they have natural beauty. We always seemed to gravitate to Colorado. To me, it is the most beautiful state. I've always said that it's God's Country.

We took a four week trip to California when Tim was eight years old. We thought we would get tired of camping, and motel it a few nights, but nope, we camped the whole time. We only had one day of rain. We went to Mesa Verde National Park in Colorado, Grand Canyon, Bryce Canyon, Zion National Park, Yosemite National Park, and many cities.

Another area we liked to visit was the Smoky Mountains National Park. Before we left home on a trip, we would make a list of animals and add to it a red barn, a yellow Volkswagen, and some such things. Then we would put a price next to each item, an amount - which we would give to the first person who saw it. A bear was worth a dollar, the rest were usually a quarter. It kept the children busy, watching the roads and hoping for some money to spend when we arrived at our destination.

When Tim was around ten years old, Paul was transferred to Des Plaines, Illinois. Beth Anne was in high school by then, Susan still in grade school. We made many good friends there, at the church and school. One family had four children, including a boy of Tim's age, named Dave. We used to all go camping together and we had a wonderful time. Dave, was so much fun, in fact the whole family was. Tim and Dave became like brothers.

The church we belonged to held a choral program the week before Christmas. Both the adult choir and the school children's choir participated, so Tim was part of the program. When we sat down, the woman in front of us turned to me and said that her two children had worked hard on their pictures, but Tim's picture had won. I told her I didn't know what she was talking about. She was amazed that I didn't know that a picture he had drawn was on the program. I was surprised too. I asked Tim later why he hadn't said anything and also that it was really nice. I don't remember what he answered, but I know now that it was because he didn't want the attention. He wanted to be like the other children, normal.

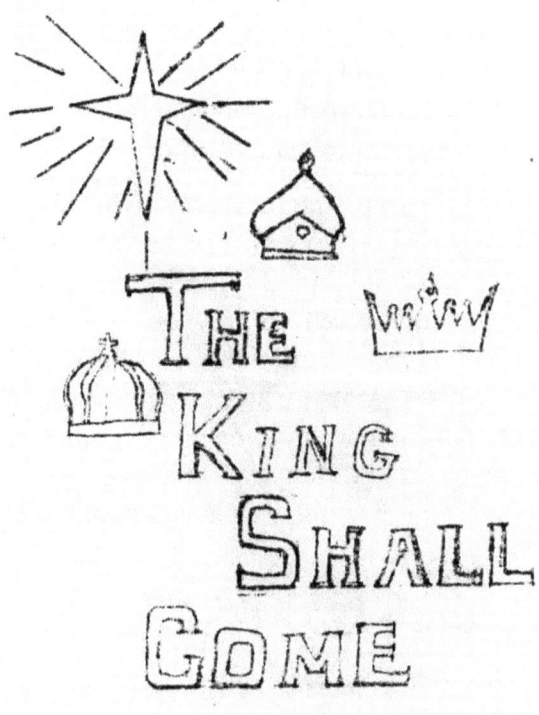

Choral Concert

Tim's design on the choral program cover

Timothy had a lot of feelings for children who were picked on, and he would speak up about it, and encourage his friends to do the same. In his seventh grade confirmation class, the religion teacher took the children across the street to the church to learn about the altar. When the teacher found one of the boys had not done his homework, she made him kneel on the marble steps for the thirty minutes the class was there. Tim did not say anything, but by his posture and snarled up face, the teacher knew he was mad. She told the principal she did not want Tim in her class anymore, and he was called into the principal's office. Tim told him he thought the boy shouldn't be punished by the teacher but by the parents. He told him it was cruel to make the boy kneel on the hard marble steps for so long. The principal agreed. Tim stayed in the class, and the school changed its rules on punishment.

Tim had always received straight A's on his report cards, but in the seventh grade he received a C in math. I asked him what was going on. He said his teacher didn't like him. I said, "Mr. West is a very dedicated teacher, he knows what you can do and you aren't doing it. I bet you are not doing your homework, are you?" He sheepishly said, no. I did not find out till many years later, when I went through his files, that he deliberately received a C so he could be like the other students. He did not like the teachers to hold him up as something special. He had never mentioned it to us. The following is a paper I found in his files that describes this event;

The Importance of Unconditional Love

The last of a generation and male, I felt the push of a clan's hopes and dreams. It was a pleasant walk for the young master. Teutonic largess and intellect belied his young age. The feminine brood of sisters, cousins, aunts and Mother teased and taunted, entertained and instructed, loved and cherished. They all were curious, even those who cursed the easy step. What the young master would become and what marvelous things he would do.

The proud Father's disciplining hand was seldom required by his progeny as he rose to challenge after challenge. The bar was simply raised. A wild temper was seemingly the only curse. His sisters exposed his Achilles heel to be his insecurities about being different and not fitting in. They paid for this knowledge as their advantage in size disappeared with time. But only a few of these tantrums were memorable; only one required stitches. His playmates seldom had the prestige to evoke such feelings or the bravery to challenge him on this lead.

School was a breeze, and he enjoyed every aspect of it. He tried everything available and always succeeded. Sports were entered without the immaturity of the gangly overgrown prince one would expect. Being just good was not really exciting anymore. He started testing the waters of failure a little at the age of eleven. The first C and maybe the first B found its way to a report card. The poor teacher who faced the challenge was the first to not find him likeable. He pushed ahead with the test to see if he could be loved as a failure. The teacher, no, the family, yes. Although he did not find the test all conclusive. He liked feeling like everyone else, but lowering his standards only accomplished this a little.

The elixir of conformity and rebellion was powerful. But he just could not be like everyone else. Even those low aspirations were attained at a different level, and he still loved success. This delicate display of personality traits and juggling of moods, of identifying with good rather than evil is still playing out.

This is the backdrop of the test he presents. The test is for unconditional love. But who can really expect this, except for perhaps from a Mother? Even then, there must be limits. Maybe it is at a less complicated level -- just the simple desire to be accepted for who he is. Not who anyone wants him to be or thinks he should be, but just for; WHO HE IS

Our last move, as a family, came at the worst possible time. Beth Anne was studying interior design, at a junior college and Susan would be going into her senior year of high school and Tim into his last year of grade school. Paul started working in Maumee, Ohio, and the children and I stayed in Des Plaines until school was out. My dad became quite ill, and he and Mom were staying with my sister Betty and her family. The children and I drove down to Indianapolis to see Dad during Easter vacation. He was going down fast, so I stayed with him the first night and the children stayed in Mom and Dad's house. I sat in a chair by his bed, helping him all night. In the morning, I went back to Mom and Dad's house to sleep and Mary Ann came to help. I had just fallen asleep when the phone rang. Dad had fallen, and they had called for an ambulance. Dad was pronounced dead at the hospital. That was very hard. We had lost Paul's parents the year before.

You most likely have figured out that Dad was very special to me and a lot of other people too. At the funeral home, a woman asked to speak to Mr. Brandt's three daughters. She told us she lived in the next block from our parents. She said she had only met Dad once and that she would never forget him. Her husband fell over dead at the lunch table one day and she called 911. My dad saw the police and ambulance down the street and walked down to see what was going on. They carried her husband out - covered, of course, - and all the emergency people drove away, leaving this woman standing by herself. Dad walked over and asked if he could help her in any way. She asked him to call her son at work and tell him what had happened. Dad went in and called her son, then stayed till the son arrived. She said Dad was so pleasant and helpful, he was like an angel sent from God to help her. We were so happy she came to tell us that. Dad had never mentioned it. To him that was just another day in his life.

Mother had dementia and couldn't stay by herself anymore, so when we moved two months later to Maumee, Ohio, Mother came and lived with us for five months, then with Mary Ann for five months, and then with Betty for five months. We three had decided that if we each had Mother for five months we would have her at different holidays. Mother went to be with Dad fifteen months after he died.

The girls finally reconciled to moving, but Tim acted as if it wasn't going to happen. Not until the moving van pulled away from our house and we got into the car to drive to Maumee, Ohio, just outside of Toledo, did he give in to the fact we were leaving. We were able to have his best friend David, from Des Plaines, come for visits that first summer, which helped. Toward the end of summer, the principal from the Lutheran school in Toledo, called to invite Tim to an eighth grade swim party at his house. We had already read about it in the bulletin, but Tim had shown no interest, because he didn't know anyone. I told the principal and he asked to speak to Tim. Afterward, Tim said he would go, but that it wouldn't be any fun. After the party, the principal said to us, "You should have been there; a few minutes after Tim arrived, the kids were yelling for him to come jump in the pool." Tim had a wonderful time. One day Tim brought a friend, Jimmy, home from school with him. Jimmy quickly told me that they had received their achievement tests back that day, and the teacher had said Tim's scores were so high they were off the scale. Jimmy said, "Tim, show your mom." Tim wasn't happy to show me, but he did. I thought he might be feeling bad, since Jimmy hadn't done as well. I see now, it was the thing about being different; he wanted to be normal. Even if we had known how much he wanted to be like the other kids, we wouldn't have fully understood it.

Tim always liked English class. He enjoyed writing stories and poems. The following is a fable Tim wrote for his eighth grade English class.

The Creature That Ate Redwoods

One day in the wild wilderness of California, an enormous monster was sighted. You have heard of Bigfoot, well, this monster made Bigfoot look like a short midget. He had the same features as Bigfoot, but was much larger. It was first sighted by Sir Trimate of England. He was rather weird and eccentric, but we should be glad that he scared away that brute of a monster.

One day when Sir Trimate was tromping through the woods, in search of who knows what. He heard a loud, strange noise. Crunch, Crunch, Crunch like the sound of someone chewing an ice cube, only louder. He peeked around the corner of a giant redwood tree, while the earth was trembling beneath his feet. He couldn't believe what he saw. There was a giant monster, picking up giant redwoods by the roots and eating them. The monster had to be at least 100 feet tall. I know, for I was an eye-witness with the strange Sir Trimate. He was wide, very wide, perhaps even 35 feet wide. Where he walked the earth shook and he left craters about the size of a PT Boat. He was strong and hairy. His hair covered his entire body. It was fire red with brown and very bristly. His face was huge and gruesome. It was fat with one large eye in the middle of his forehead.

He saw Trimate and picked him up; he tried to eat him just as we would eat a small piece of candy. I previously reported that ole' Sir Trimate scared the big brute away. Well, he did, in a very unusual way. When the monster tried to eat Trimate, he was scared stiff by the taste of this strange human. Ole Trimate hadn't taken a bath for over ten years and had a very foul taste.

The monster, shocked by this, ran back to his home in hell. The whole time he was yelling that his eternal torture in Hades was better than the taste or looks of Ole' Sir Trimate.

You have heard of San Francisco. Boy, that is what the brute left behind him when he blundered back home. He also caused the fault line in California and cleared out a great number of redwood trees, too.

Note: As a fable, the moral of this story is------Never take a bath, just in case you are met by your neighborhood monster.

Tim was chosen valedictorian of his eighth grade class. One of the mothers was upset because her daughter wasn't chosen, so she went to the principal and complained. Her reasoning was that Tim had only been there one year and her daughter had been there a few years longer. She was informed it was given to the person with the higher scores. I was surprised that she would do something like that.

Timothy was very athletic and while in grade school played basketball and ran track. Quite often, he would play tennis with the principal and his wife at the park.

3

Tim's High School and College Years

When he went into high school, Tim added football to his sports. His grades were still excellent, even with all of the high school activities. When he turned sixteen, he found a job at a pancake restaurant close by our house. He started out busing tables and then became a waiter. Tim liked to cook and became a good one.

There was one time that he had problems with a teacher, his English teacher during his junior year. She had a reputation of picking on a student every year. I guess Tim was it, that year. She didn't think an athlete should be taking advanced placement classes. She always verbally tore Tim's work apart and Tim would try to defend himself. I remember she once gave him an F on a paper he had written, because she said he plagiarized it. The book he had used was loaned him by another teacher. He brought it in to prove he hadn't copied it. The paper mentioned ammunition being stored in magazines and the teacher laughed "in periodicals" she asked. Tim and I went to the school principal to get that one straightened out.

Our home was busy during Tim's high school years. He had a girlfriend whom we all liked. He went with her for almost four years. We enjoyed his friends, nice young men. If they were at our home when we were about to eat, we set a place for them at the table. I remember going to a basketball game at the high school and yelling for Tim when he made a basket. A woman in front of me turned around and asked, "Is Tim your son?" I said yes, and she said she had been a substitute teacher in his French class that day. She wanted me to know what a nice and polite young man he was. Of course, being his mother, I was very happy to hear that.

Until this time we had seen no indication of any mental problems. The one big problem with Tim, at this time, was that he had started drinking and he didn't seem to be able to stop. I talked and talked to him about it. He would agree with me, and I would have hope that he would quit, but no such luck. Paul said all boys usually try it, and he would stop. I didn't agree. He had a stronger draw to it than his friends. Paul and I were not drinkers. Paul would have a beer if someone came over, I might have a glass of wine on rare occasions, and that was it.

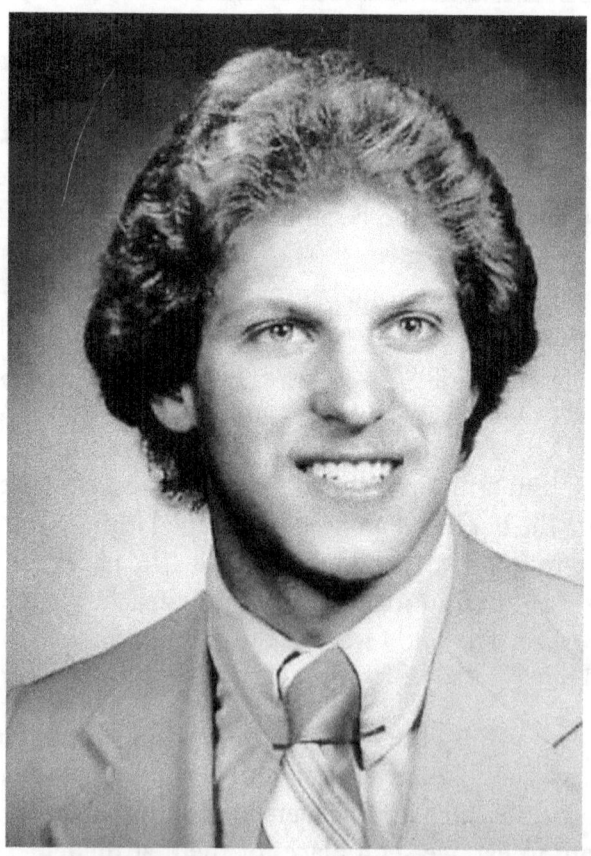

Timothy Brandt Niemann 1982 senior picture

Tim was accepted into Purdue University's engineering program. When he came home for Christmas break, I had arranged that he and I would talk with a counselor at one of the hospitals. The counselor thought it was great that Tim and I were addressing his drinking before any police problems had arisen. Tim agreed with me that he should stop drinking, but he seemed to think he could have one, like his friends, and stop with that, - but he couldn't.

On a spring break from Purdue in 1983, Tim went to visit friends at Bowling Green State University. He was stopped by a state trooper, arrested, and released. Charges were reduced from a DUI "to impaired with DUI." He had to attend a course and pay a thousand - dollar fine. Tim only attended Purdue for one year. He said he was not happy there; none of his friends were there. For his second year, he went to Ohio University in Athens, Ohio.

As well as Tim's main 40 page journal, Susan and I found folders, where he had all of his police encounters listed - all the rehabs he had attended - court papers - letters and drawings from his three nieces - his thoughts - phrases he especially liked - cards from people he liked. We were amazed how Tim had kept everything so neatly filed away, and his life was in such chaos. The following was one of Tim's police encounters.

I had recently broke up with a girl I had dated for almost 4 years and was severely depressed and broke out in crying sprees. All I could do was drink. I went to a big dance club to drink and have fun. When I left there, I was quickly arrested. sentenced to 10 days; 3 days in jail and 7 in work release.

That was in the winter of 1984. Paul and I didn't know about Tim's crying sprees and depression. We knew he was a little down about breaking up with his girlfriend. It was always Tim and I who went through all these things. I was available, and of course Paul was at work. Paul is a sweet man, but I believe he was hiding his head in the sand so he didn't have to face it. It is hard to admit when there is a problem. I wanted so much for Tim to be able to straighten up. I loved Tim so, and I wanted him to succeed in life. There didn't seem to be anyone I could talk openly to about Tim. Our pastor asked me one morning how Tim was doing. I told him that I had given up, that Tim was never going to change. He told me that perhaps if jail was not going to help Tim, maybe him being there would help someone else. Tim called me from jail the next day and told me he was teaching a Bible study class there. When I saw the pastor, I told him that he was right, that Tim may be helping someone else.

By this time Paul and I were beside ourselves. This brilliant son of ours was out of control. I talked and talked to Tim. He would agree that he should stop drinking; he just was not able to do it. It was so frustrating. We had so many hopes and dreams for him, and he did too. His sister Susan and I sat him down and talked to him about what he was doing to himself and the whole family. He would look so sad, and he wouldn't say much except that he was sorry. He said, "Mom, I am not doing this to hurt you. I just don't know why I can't stop, the way others do." Susan and I would feel so sorry for him. He never argued with us, no matter what we said to him. He would look so sad.

For a time I was so embarrassed and down in the dumps, I stopped going to church. Everyone knew him and would ask, "what's Tim doing"? I certainly didn't want to say, "Oh, he is in jail." One weekend, my nephew Chris drove up from Indianapolis to see Susan and her husband. He stopped to see Paul and me too. When he went home, I received a call from my sister Betty. She wanted to know if there was something wrong. Chris told her, "Aunt Carol is really different, she is real quiet and not fun anymore." Well, that was all it took for me to wake up and see what I was doing to myself, my family, and most importantly to my Lord and Savior. I went to church the next Sunday and have continued to this day. Thank you, Christopher, for getting me back on the right track.

In the fall of 1986, Police thought I looked suspicious walking home at 3:00 A.M. stopped me and found .25 ounce of marijuana and took me to jail. Fined $30.

By this time, all Tim needed to graduate with his engineering degree was one quarter of college. He never was able to go back and get it. He tried several times, but couldn't stay sober. It looked to me as if he didn't want to straighten up. I told him he could no longer live with us. He was working at the Red Lobster restaurant and moved in with a couple of fellow workers. He went almost a year without seeing us or calling. I started having medical problems, a pain here or there. The doctor would have me get an x-ray or some test and the nurse would call and say,

"Good news, they couldn't find anything". I would tell her, I still have the pain. I told the doctor that I felt like a hypochondriac. Finally I ended up in the hospital with an asthma attack. Paul called and left Tim a message at his apartment. Tim called me in the hospital and we talked, and when I came home he did stop over. Tim was such a fine human being when he wasn't drinking or smoking pot. That is why it was so hard dealing with his behavior. I didn't understand how my child could be so far off the right path. It was not until 1987 that he went into a substance abuse facility for 30 days in Toledo.

Entered my first treatment program at 24. It was strongly suggested by my Mother that I enlist. I did not understand much about alcoholism, just that I liked it better drunk. I completed the 30 day program and stayed sober another 45 days. It felt so good to drink again.

In the fall of 1989, I took my girl friend to Bowling Green for her birthday. We got very drunk and then made it to her house. Decided we needed to get to town for cigarettes and I was arrested. Sentenced to 6 months in Work Release. Got fired and was remanded to the work

House for the remainder.

This must be the time that Tim wrote the forty page journal, Susan and I found in his files, after his death.

4

Tim's Journal

October 8

Days in jail do not pass fast, even if you are trying to make the best of them. I am trying to look back over my life to find my strengths and weaknesses, likes and dislikes, passions and abhorrences, and my beliefs and perceptions of how it is. My goal in all this: to find a career path which leads to areas of my greatest enjoyment and fulfillment and stays within the boundaries of my beliefs in good and evil.

My strengths lie in areas of analysis, problem solving, and being fair. Being able to look at a situation and objectively discerning the maximum solution. I am athletic and have stamina. When my interest is kept, I can work on a project for a long time.

I enjoy sports of all types. I especially enjoy the NFL and I like to play basketball, golf, fish, and football. I love computer games and enjoy finding applications for their use. I am interested in the World and want to see it. Learning peoples customs and beliefs is very interesting. Along with this is my passion for history, politics and economics.

We'll get back to this kind of thing later; now, on to things of a more current nature, how I feel and what I think now. My aspirations are to find happiness, love and peace. I feel that I can do this by pursuing my interests, pray to God, and by not letting my fears dictate my actions.

October 9

Today has been a tough day for me. Realizing that I could be in here until March seems unbelievable, but all too real. After breakfast I took a nice nap, talked for a while, and then went to lunch. We played cards, the normal group; a game of spades for soup. It all ended even. I went to the Chemical Dependency Group where we watched a video on violence and alcohol. Now that I have been to a few of these type classes, I know what a joke they are. Why are they bothering. It seems very unlikely that they could help anyone.

The faith I am developing in God keeps me going through these times. I just haven't felt very social today, but I have been trying. I thank God for Dan, even though he drives me nuts sometimes, his humor and outlook, but most of all his easy extension of himself, keeps me feeling like a human. I know God has His purpose for me, and that these trials give me a chance to grow, but I want to get out of here. As Dan pointed out to me, I haven't done much to get out. I think he is right and I'm going to spend sometime writing to the Judge and my lawyer this weekend. I talked to my father this evening. I was kind of short with him, and I feel bad about it. I was terribly grumpy and I could barely hear him and was a little discouraged to find out that no one has contacted my lawyer. But hey, this is my mess. And hey, I have quit smoking and I am closer to God than I ever have been. I want to stay close to God and start following my heart.

The interesting part of the day has been an old man from Portage, Ohio who is writing letters to 20/20 and the jail director about the horrible conditions here. I wish him luck, but his ranting has been pure comedy. He is quite upset about the horrible food and the fact that women C.O.'s walk in the shower and bathroom facilities. He is new to this kind of thing and I'm sure he will realize his position soon.

It is almost bed time now and I will try to express my feelings:

A person falls into many circumstances, he

usually doesn't know why.

I have come to realize I don't have to keep falling,

or know the reasons why.

The trick is to do the things that please you,

in the most unselfish way.

To believe in God's existence and that He really

wants you to play.

I don't exactly understand what has happened to

my ambition,

Has fear of failure harnessed all my dreams?

Why can't I make a decision, a plan?

October 10

Providence has finally stricken me with a simple honest hit delivered by a hippie. That divine intervention I have been waiting for to show me how to serve God and how to make a living isn't going to come. It took the honest words of a Dan to tell me that I am not that damn special. I have to grab what I want and not worry about if its right or if it is what my family or friends want. I will earn their respect by being successful at what I like to do. My goal list has been begun. I am making a list of everything I want to accomplish and like to do as these things occur to me. It is a short list now, but it will grow, as I do. I have decided to take an active role in my quest for freedom. I am going to try the impossible. Hopefully well written letters to the Judge and lawyer can help with an early release. I am also going to try to acquire a job from within these walls. Work release would be a welcome deliverance from here. God is finally working in me.

Today is bright. I sure want to get out of here, but that isn't going to get me down. Dan showed me another passage in the A.A. Big Book that rang home. It involved a fellow who ws miserable in the program because he couldn't take the first step. I am sure that this applies to me, but I am still not sure I am going back to A.A.

October 11

It was football day, the best day in jail. I woke up feeling pretty good, had a lovely breakfast of grits, bread, a hard boiled egg, and an orange. I went to church and listened to three women preach. I really enjoy these non-denominational preachers who teach out of the Bible. It fills my soul with joy and gives me hope. Some of my friends here criticize me a little bit because they say people will grab onto anything in jail and then forget it as soon as they get out.

I look at it like this. The last time I was in jail I was so convinced it was unjust, I wanted to prove that it wouldn't do me any good by not letting it, and it didn't. This time I am doing everything that will make me a better person, and church and reading the Bible are tops on my list. I think I offended Dan when I told him I was surprised that he didn't go to church and that church was the best thing in here because the CCNO staff didn't have anything to do with it. He retorted that it was the same with A.A., "but A.A. sucks," I said, referring to the meeting in here.

There was a lot of talk about the fact that the Judge doesn't let anyone out today. A lot of people are getting out of this dorm soon and I guess that inspires talk. I am not going to get discouraged though and am going to do whatever I can. Dan has been down since he realized 10 days wasn't going to be enough for him. He got some decent news today, I thought, about a decent chance he will be out in 30. I wish I had got that, but he is still being pissey. Just the in and out and pros and cons of being locked up.

I am more convinced than ever that I finally got my head on straight. I don't feel sorry for myself at all about being in here or my past problems. I think a lot of my problems stem from trying to be something I am not. I always thought I had to do something great. Now I just feel that I have to do something well. It really takes a lot of pressure off and I can't wait to put it into practice. I have been doing things I thought I should or feeling guilty about not doing them for years and never realized it. I don't know exactly what happened to me, but I feel great.

October 12

It has been a pretty uneventful day. I slept a lot because I couldn't last night for some reason. I played a game of Risk; I was the first one out. After talking briefly to my lawyer last night, I sent him a letter telling him to get me out of here today. I started feeling kind of stupid about coming in here today. I probably should have taken off at least until the Judge retired. Oh, well, that's the price you pay for not being in charge of your life. I hope I never let my family's thoughts dictate my actions again.

It has been uplifting to see my bunky, James, get caught up in the spirit of reform. He is a nice guy, kind of simple, and has been apparently messing around for awhile. He has started to participate in my and Dan's conversations and is also trying to make constructive plans upon release. I hope they work out for him.

My faith in God keeps my spirits high, even when my optimism fades. I truly believe something good is going to happen to me. I pray it involves leaving this place. I seem to be learning more about myself every day and getting more comfortable with it. I feel so ambitious.

October 13

Fifteen days into this sentence, it's kind of hard to believe. The time's going by all right, but I can't imagine 4 1/2 more months!! For some reason the laundry person didn't come by today and all my whites are dirty. We got to play basketball today and I finally played halfway decent. It is hard to play wearing glasses, but my eyes are finally starting to get used to them. I also told the counselor to put me on a list to go in the trustee dorm.

I am disappointed that I have not received any mail. Everyone says they are going to write, it kind of pisses me off. I thought someone might send money too, but here I am going on three weeks and zilch. Oh well, I refuse to get resentful or feel sorry for myself, and the wonderful thing about that is I really don't. I sure don't feel like I deserve this sentence, but I sure knew it was possible. I am going to fight any way I can to get out of here.

I went to a neat Church Service tonight. We watched a video of a speaker who talked about God's Word being the truth and that the truth brings trust. We should be true to our word and then we earn trust and believe in ourselves. This makes a lot of sense. Also, I am starting to learn and be able to feel great. I don't know where these feelings come from except from God, and that makes it easy to believe. I pray that I get out of here, and with God's help, I will.

I played Monopoly with the boys after I got back from Church. It was fun, but I can't win. That smart ass hippie wins every time. And poor James doesn't quite have a broker's mentality, so you got to try to rip him off before someone else does. It came as no surprise that our gypsy friend is a good business man. He has had quite the interesting life, even if he has spent way too much of it behind bars. He provided us with some good entertainment tonight. As James went to put some soup in the microwave, one of the Mexicans told him to f--- off in Spanish, not thinking we understood, because he wanted to use the microwave. The gypsy jack, understood Spanish. So when James came back to the table, he told James to say "I f--- your Mother, bitch," in Spanish, not thinking James would say it clear enough or loud enough to be understood. Wrong!! The little Mexican was quite offended. James looked pretty funny when he realized he had been duped.

I still don't know what to think about A.A. and all that. I want to live according to God, and I want to enjoy life. I hate putting so much effort into not doing something and that's what I feel like I am doing in A.A. I am going to try to keep my priorities focused, striving towards goals, and see what happens. I think I will do fine. Pot is another sticky situation. Sometimes I like it, sometimes it makes me worthless. I will have to watch myself. I think I am going to find I don't need it anymore.

October 15

I talked to Russ and Rachael tonight. They were very encouraging and happy to hear from me. It was great to talk to them. I feel very good about myself and I feel loved. I am full of ambition and am getting anxious in here. It is just very frustrating to see people with such dramatically smaller sentences for the same crime. I want out of here and I am going to keep working at it.

I am encouraged with the progress I have made towards getting into work release. God must be smiling on me. I have sent in a request to see Sheila Blank, Russ's mothers friend, for further assistance. My case manager is just unresponsive and pathetic. I hope things are progressing with Judge Blank. I sent him a letter just in case.

I feel the legal profession may be for me. That is what I used to want to do and I chose a different path for silly reasons. I don't know how realistic it is for me to make such a change now, but I sure like the idea. Maybe Aubrey will be good for something. When I talked to Russ, he said Aubrey wanted to help. I am going to try to get hold of him.

It seems to me that the corruption of our present society and the corruption of our legal system are not independent occurrences. The judges have become criminals and criminals judges; woe to those who fall in between. When the Court House becomes a source of revenue, corruption flows out into every crack of society. If the crime is common, it is too much trouble to deal with. If revenues can be brought in, it must be the scourge of civilization. This is the premise of our common law.

October 16

This has been a down day for me. It started off when the little weasel known as "what the f_ _ _ ", because of his nasal intonation of his favorite phrase, started telling me about Judge Blank. I told him he was full of shit. He retorted, "why would I lie," and I responded, "because you're a little weaselly ass liar." He had no reply. I had no intention of letting that little festering creature insinuate anything about my intelligence.

I then went to a chemical dependency class where I received another dose insufferable bullshit. I am edgy today these stupid things are driving me nuts. No one cares anything about what happens in the program and it is just as stupid for me to attend.

I have been trying to attain some peace with God today, but it just won't come. I want to get out of here so bad, and I just don't understand why I should be here so long. I haven't been able to go to Church all week, that will certainly help. I can't wait to see my parents Sunday. I hope they will try to get me out of here. I am going to call Aubrey tonight and see what he can do.

October 17

I was unexpectedly moved to the trustee dorm last night. I don't know how this was accomplished so quick. I had to get up at 5 in the morning to begin my duties. I am on the A.M. kitchen crew and spent my time washing pots and pans. It certainly isn't a fun job, but it wasn't that bad. I only have to do it until someone new is moved to our crew. This should happen within a few days.

I was kind of nervous about leaving my familiar surroundings, but everything is going fine. There are a lot of nice people in here, quite a few goof balls, but no one threatening. I have not found my peer group yet; that will come. I do get to eat well and I think time will go a lot faster with a job. I tried to watch football today, but I ended up napping, then ate dinner and went to Church.

After a tough day yesterday, God has brought me back to his peace. I must remember that no matter what I do, I am a man of God and he will forgive me. I know He exists, because of the way he makes me feel when I am near him. My life is getting clearer and clearer for me. I know now that I am a business man. I know I want to become a lawyer also. I have thought about it for some time and it still seems attractive. I am going to pray on it tonight. I do not feel afraid to leap into life and take some chances; I trust God.

October 18

Getting up at 5 in the morning is still hard on me. I sleep a lot now but always feel tired. I just have not got into the new routine yet and found the in and outs in the kitchen. My diet has improved, but it can get a lot bet ter. The Higgs had a Church Service for us today. They are such happy people and bring a powerful message. I always feel very uplifted after hearing them preach.

My Mother and Father came to visit today. I had been waiting with much anticipation and it was great to see them. I was kind of grumpy because of lack of sleep, but very much enjoyed the visit. I stressed some of the bad points of this institution and my great desire to leave here. I hope I did not upset them, but I have to be sure they are trying to get me out.

I tried to watch football after the visit, but was too tired. I did see that my NFL team is still doing well. I now have the 1st and 3rd running backs as well as a great tandem of running backs. I miss my friends from K-100 and still haven't replaced them in here yet. It is kind of nice to have some time to myself to read and write again though. I have been reading a book about the Russion Revolution and the Bible. God has given me some inspiration in my need to write Judge Blank and I plan on working on that tonight. I will keep asking for help.

October 19

Things are starting to smooth out for me in my new surroundings. I got to play basketball with the brothers today and had a good time. They played a surprisingly good brand of hoops. My sleeping is still messed up, and if not for a big kind - hearted brother named Ron, I would have missed my work detail the last two days. Hopefully I will sleep tonight even though I napped today. The last 3 days I have spent here have flown by. There were some new arrivals tonight, so I am done doing pots and pans. My next job will be a lot easier.

I have made much progress on getting into work release lately, but I am keeping at it and have acquired an application. Tomorrow I will meet my new case worker and hopefully things will progress.

I feel very good still and can't wait to get into the world. I am confident things will go well for me. My new understanding of living my own life has brought new life to me and I thank God. For many years I thought the things I wanted were the things others wanted for me or the things others wanted. Russ and Rachel are planning a visit for a week from Saturday and I am anxious to see them. I hope I am out by then, but I know it is very possible I won't be.

October 20

Today went by very well. I finally got some sleep last night and was able to get up for work without Ron getting me up. The brothers asked me to be on their basketball team, what an honor. I met my new case manager and found her quite agreeable. I think I am making progress in getting into work release. After Church, I called Aubrey in the hopes that he may be able to help me get out. I have to talk to him tomorrow afternoon. I finally got an easy job doing dishes in the kitchen, so my job is much more pleasant.

I wrote judge Blank a letter trying to get out. I prayed for help in writing it and I received it through sudden inspiration. I am trying to let God run my life and I think I am learning how. I just keep trying. At Church, we watched a video from the 'Christian Men's Network' with Edwin Louis Cole. He talked about how God's Word is his bond to us. Since we are in God's likeness, our word is our bond to others. In other words, be true to your word and you will be true to yourself. I can't wait to get out of here, but I feel very good. I still think I want to be an attorney.

October 21

I am kind of anxious today. I have been doing a lot of reading, but my right shoulder is so sore, it prevents me from lying on it for very long. The muscle and nerve are pinched, just like from football. I guess it is from doing pushups, so I quit doing them. I talked to Aubrey today and he was going to contact Richard to see what could be done for me. I also mailed my letter to Judge Blank today and am praying to God to provide a miracle for me. The thought of staying here until March terrorizes me. I sure hope something works out for me. I can't believe I still feel sure I want to be a lawyer, but I have been neglecting my work on plans for the future. I do know of things I want to pursue (listed on goal page) and I know I have to find some kind of job, make some headway on my bills, get car registered, and hopefully get driving privileges. These all seem like goals I can accomplish within a month.

I am trying to think back to see if I have ever been so relaxed and confident about my future. I really feel that I have some direction and that most of all, it is entirely derived from within myself. I think most people would consider it a little absurd to pursue a career in law at this point in my life. I know that it would serve many purposes for me. I would like being a lawyer in itself, but it may also open up doors into politics for me. Also, it would allow me to work for myself, and most of all, a chance to right some of the wrongs I feel most passionate about.

October 22

It has been a strange day here at CCNO. I was finally getting used to my trustee schedule, when I was moved to a new dorm after my shift today. When I first arrived here, I had filled out an application to get into the "New Beginnings Program," a substance abuse program. But after getting acclimated to my situation. I told my case manager that I was no longer interested in it and wanted to go to the trustee dorm, (3 weeks ago). She never withdrew my application and I was moved here today.

Shortly after I moved, Pastor came out to visit. We had a nice talk. I told him that I was reading the Bible and about some of the changes going on in my life. He was very supportive. I told him I wanted to become a lawyer and he told me his son had just become one, doing it kind of late in life. Then I went to Church; it was the Catholic's night. There is one man there who has taken an interest in me. He always tells me I have a good attitude. That inspires me; I talked about my views on what Jesus meant about poverty. I said that the amount of money is not what is important, but it is to realize that it did not come from us. Humble does not mean wimpy, it means a realistic view of who we are in the scheme of things. That is not to belittle us or to praise ourselves. We are both sinners and saints. As often as we sin, which is often, we are renewed through God's grace and forgiveness.

I also may have received my first write up tonight. It will be interesting to see. The CO in this dorm is a real punk. After Church I told him that my white clothes were coming from the laundry to L1, my old dorm. Eventually he brought a bag and dumped them on me and my bed. I continued reading. When I went to fold them up, I noticed that socks were missing. I went to inform him that I needed 2 pair of socks and he responded, "Well you're not getting them from me." I said, "Well can't you call someone?". He replied, "Who do you want me to call, the director?' This sordid little affair continued till I turned around and said, "F _ _ _ you," under my breath. Then he threatened to write me up. I walked away. I certainly will fight that, I should win.

I have decided that I am not going to pursue AA immediately after my release. I need to keep writing my feelings, praying, and reading the Bible. I will figure out where drinking and pot fit into my life, if at all. I need to start making plans for my release. I have some ideas, as stated before. I should be able to get unemployment and I want to live with Russ and Rachael again. I have not heard anything from Beth yet, but I would like to at least visit them. I hope I hear from her soon.

October 23

Well, I moved back tonight and I didn't get written up, Cool! It has been a very boring day and I am glad to be moved back to the trustee dorm. Hopefully I will get my old job back. I spent the day reading Genghis Khan. I'm going to read some more and go to bed. I just haven't been very motivated today.

The journey begins without directions

I march and march along the path.

Some is trodden, some is swath.

Changing scenes, moods and complexions.

Experience is the source of feelings,

Collectively or on our own.

Grinding teeth and broken bones,

Grow into joy without a ceiling.

Finally directions are revealed,

Not from a man though, from within.

The spirit entered is the engine,

Giving faith to follow the willed.

The hearts desires seem too a far.

October 24

It is funny how your moods change. Today everthing went very well. I feel very close to God and feel that, with Him, I can endure anything. The Church service I went to was great. A black couple from Defiance came in and they are always great. He taught that the only thing we can offer God is praise. Church is our chance to commune and praise God. We need to pursue God everyday. I have come to an understanding of this.

One cannot live another man's morality. I must follow my heart. I do this through prayer and staying in touch with my feelings, this is how I talk to God. That is what makes drug abuse sinful, it inhibits our ability to stay in contact wih God by offering up our feelings. I know that I can withstand staying in jail the entire 6 months now, but I feel very strongly that God has other plans. I will not be overly disappointed if I am wrong though. I am not quite sure how things turned around for me, but I no longer feel ashamed, embarrassed or that I have anything to prove. I am confident, though, that good things are in store for me no matter what is put in front of me. I want to live to the Glory of God.

My upper back is killing me for some reason. I have to have it looked at when I get out of here. It seems to be related to a football injury I received 11 years ago. Every time I lift weights or do push ups, I have to watch it. But I quit push ups almost 2 weeks ago and it still hurts. Mom and Jennifer are coming tomorrow. Always great to see them; I love them so much. It is painful to see them though, for it reminds me of all the reasons I want out of here so bad.

October 25

I had a nice visit with Mom and Jennifer. Susan and Rick will be gone before I get out. Slept most of the day because my back hurts too much to do anything else. Talked to Russ. He and Rachael will be out next Sunday. Made it to Church today. Back hurts too much to think about writing.

October 27

Ah, relief. My back is a little tight, but the soreness is gone. Prayer works. I have changed the position I sleep in and the nurse came and rubbed Ben-Gay on my back last night. Also the guard told me that Tylenol actually loosens the muscles. All of these things resulted in a much happier back today.

This work release thing seems to be progressing very well. Judge Blank faxed the O.K. for HIT program on Monday. I had Linda call over to the Work Release people that afternoon which netted me a conference with Joe Lamb later that day. Today I had an interview with the man who runs the factory and Joe said things seemed to go well. I told him a little about myself; why I am here, education, work experience, how long I'll be here. Hopefully I will be over there this week. The job entails working with mentally and emotionally handicapped people in a pallet factory. I will make a whopping $4.25 hr., but I can't wait. It just seems like things are working out for me.

I played basketball pretty well today with my new back, nearly beating the brothers in a game of 21. I also played football where I intercepted a pass. A good day at rec. I am starting to fit in well in this dorm. I get along well with the black guys I work with and have fun listening to their stories about life in the "jungle." These have led me to some new insights into myself and about life in general. I have a new confidence about me.

You cannot follow another man's morality, just as you cannot live in two worlds. This leaves a person listless and scrambling to survive. Eventually his unstable footing fails him and he falls. You have to follow your own heart. It leads you to happiness. Feelings cannot discern the truth. Sometimes they point toward spiritual desires, sometimes physical; they cannot be relied upon for decision making. When you follow your heart, you are not guaranteed of making the best decision making. When you follow your heart, you are not guaranteed of making the best decision, but you are guaranteed to make a good decision.

I am still very hypercritical of myself and I have got to straighten this out. As I become more and more involved with the Bible and my faith, I find myself again holding myself to impossible standards. I must remember to be content with heading in the right direction, happy with small gains, aware of my humanness. Ah, this is the key. As I strive for godliness, I have to remember my humanness without condemning myself. I need to be aware of when my desires are leading me away from the direction I want to head. Of course I will desire woman, booze, etc. And even if I act on these desires, it does not mean I am not a Christian, just human. The idea is to stay in touch with God and keep on learning. God wants me to enjoy life, but he wants me to begin enjoying the things he enjoys. I am going to start doing at least one nice thing every day. A kind word, help with a problem, some consolation. Today I wrote a letter to Judge Blank for a Puerto Rican guy, who does not write English very well. He wants to get in the HIT program with me. I really don't have to try to do these things because I want to.

October 28

I still have not heard anything about work release, but I am still hopeful. I expected to receive Judge Blanks answer to my letter, but I did not see it either. My spirits are remaining high and life is going along. Today is my one month anniversary. A month in jail is a long time. I tried to trim my beard today and made a mess of it. I didn't do my hair a lot of good either.

The excitement of the day was a game of flag football. I cracked heads with a guy in here and really messed him up. I hope he is OK. We were both going for the quarterback from opposite sides and my forehead hit him right under the eye. It swelled up a lot and left a slit about an inch long. He was dazed and probably has a concussion. My head is sore and I slept the afternoon away, but I think I am fine. We did win by the way.

My back seems to be fine and I even did push ups again. It is still a little stiff, but I keep at it. I went to Bible study tonight. Pat and Ron, two guys in my dorm, have started it and we three go together for some fellowship. We read Galatians five and talked about listening to the Spirit. Learning to pay attention to that inner voice. I stressed to them my belief in learning through our experiences. Conforming our lives to the Bible in ways that let the Spirit take care of our problems. The importance of not condemning ourselves, but to stay in the right direction. That is what is important. My reoccurring theme again. We must live our own morality. Our convictions must emanate from within ourselves even if they don't originate there. They must make sense to us and have meaning to us. God wants me to be happy.

I have made great strides in determining what I want to do with my life. Now, I need to spend some time making my plans more concrete. I know that I want to be a lawyer. I am going to aim at becoming a trial lawyer with the aim of one day becoming a State Senator. But first things first. I have to decide how I am going to apply as a bartender at places immediately. I think this is smart because it will leave days open to look for real work or to work with Russ. That is my other thoughts. I am going to convince Russ to form some sort of partnership and I am going to actively pursue work. I will leave him behind if that is what he wants. I have often been very passive and I am through with that. We should be able to make a lot of money power washing and need to find large painting jobs where we can hire a crew. It is time to be responsible for success or failure.

Next I must decide where I want to live. I have a bag of feelings on this matter and I don't have anything concrete to go on. This is why I would like to visit Beth and Susan when I get out. I also think I would enjoy Florida. If I move, I must do it soon so I establish residency for school. I kind of feel that will move at the beginning of summer.

October 29

Things went well today, although I started off slow. After sleeping off my concussion yesterday afternoon, I did not sleep well last night. I was a little down this morning and really wanted to get out of here. Then at about 10:30 A.M. I was called from work to go to the doctor to check my back. He said I had some strained muscles and to take it easy and take some Motrin. While I was there, the nurse asked me if I was going to work release. I told her I had been trying to arrange that, but did not know for sure. She kind of let it slip that there was something to that effect in my file. I expected to go over there tonight; hopefully, I will go in the morning.

I have not called Aubrey or got my response back from judge Blank. I was hoping for the letter from the Judge so I could tell if my change in status was due solely from the letters I wrote. The timing indicates that it was. If this is so, I am really going to get on Richard to do something to earn his money. He knew what my circumstance was when I entered his counsel and he led me to believe he could help me. For a thousand dollars, I should get something, and I plan on letting him know that. I am going to work on a draft to him tonight and then pray to God for guidance. I will rewrite it over the weekend and send it out Monday. I think I will call Aubrey tomorrow afternoon and see if he has come across anything.

October 30

Another day over. I was kind of pissy today, but I seemed to make the right conciliations and things turned out all right. I am just very anxious to get out. You never really get used to being in jail, but you do learn to make it bearable. My trust in God goes a long way toward achieving that result.

The Bible Study tonight revolved around the troubles and trials we have and why God allows them to happen. Ron, an older gentleman, who has a drinking problem, is very upset about how his life is going and how his wife is treating him. I keep telling him he has to live for himself. Trust God in that what is happening is for a reason, no matter how absurd it seems, and to thank God for it, for everything. I now understand what living for yourself is all about. I have decided that it is important that I start thinking about all the little things I want. I have finally discovered that this is where our sense of direction comes from. And the methods we use to acquire these ends depend upon our character and convictions. These ends and means are in a continuous feed back loop and are the manifestation of the person we are or are not. I know I want a place to live where I can live as I choose. The necessity, freedom, and joy of driving outweigh the risks and I will move to reduce those risks as quickly as possible. I need enough money to have some security. I am tired of blowing in the wind. I want a girlfriend. I want to become a lawyer. I want to find a job that allows me to have these things. I want to begin acquiring some material things. I want to stay in touch with God. I need to make a decision about a Church.

October 31

Church tonight confirmed my feelings of being on the right track. I know my quest for spiritualness in itself will make me a better and happier person. It seems that Christians are constantly speaking of suffering and

I think they are missing something. It was the search for happiness itself that brought me back to God. The suffering in his behalf is not truly suffering. The teacher tonight seemed to share my belief in letting God tell you what to do. Sins are sins in that they lead you from the path. One man's morality need not match another's. I think that is the essence of God's grace.

I can not wait to see Russ and Rachael tomorrow. I am glad my beard looks good again. I have heard that the Judge got another D.U.I. I must find out if it is true. I am going to make sure this story gets out if it is. The man is clearly insane. I wonder what makes him do what he does. Maybe I will get out because of this somehow. I am going to keep working on getting out. I thought this effort would drive me crazy, but I am quite at peace.

My friend Ron found out his wife is serving him with divorce papers. He is holding up well, although he says he is dying inside. He must learn to live for himself. Self control is as important as self-esteem, I am finding. And this self control must not be derived from fear of repercussions, but on the knowledge that it will yield better things. That is the secret. That is why our goals must be derived internally.

I have heard some encouraging things about getting out. With the election tomorrow, it is only a matter of time till Judge Blank will be out of office. Along with this, I have heard that he is before a review board. Also, it is rumored that he got a D.U.I. recently. I do not know how many of these things are true, but it gives me encouragement and makes me think that he will be out of office soon. One of the guys that I never thought would be released early by Judge Blank is out. He had served only little more of his six month sentence than I. Things are going to happen for me.

I talked to Mom, Susan and Jennifer on the phone. Things seem to be going well for them. I don't think they know quite what to think of me now. I know they see a curious change. And the great thing about it is that I don't care if they approve. Not in a negative way, but because I know I want good things. I also got my student loan deferred until March hopefully. Mom had to do a little footwork for me and hopefully that was completed. I am going to call Russ and Aubrey tomorrow and see if there is any news. Supposedly, Russ is coming out Wednesday. Maybe he will come with Aubrey.

I played a little basketball at rec. today. I played alright but my shooting isn't there and I am awful wimpy offense for some reason. I am starting to really get along well with the people in the dorm. I can't believe I am not over in work release yet, but things are cool. I am going to try and get out of the kitchen soon, I am tired of it already.

November 3

Clinton is the President. Hurrah!! America has a chance. It has been another good day for me. I talked to Russ today and he is coming for a visit tomorrow. He will hopefully bring news about the Judge and my chances for release.

I did not sleep a lot last night and I was kind of grumpy today at work. I have got to work on that. I can become so belligerent and make such a big deal of little things sometime. Leonard, the Supervisor, asked Cassidy, who looks like Jim from "Taxi", to bring some trays back to the dish area and I got kind of stupid about it. I played ball and lifted weights which was cool.

I went to the Christian Men's Network tonight. A very nice person named Clancy brings us videos and talks to us. It is always very interesting, educational and inspirational. The topic tonight was the uniqueness of woman. Edwin Allen Holt spoke of things of the masculine and feminine. He talked about how a woman needs to feel unique in order to submit to a man. A woman and God both want the same three things from a man: consistency, decisiveness, and strength. I continue to learn in here everyday. God keeps my outlook positive and helps me to learn in all things. I have been reading Revelations and it has been slow going. It is interesting but very hard to understand. It sounds like Christ is going to set up a kingdom on Earth. I think I will have to read this book many times. Tomorrow I am going to write Beth again. I hope I get a response from her. I may also write to the Blade about Judge Blank. I sure hope Russ brings me some news.

November 4

It is late and I must get to bed, but I wanted to make an entry. I wrote Beth a letter telling her what I have been up to. Russ visited but didn't have much news. I hope Aubrey can find some information out for me. Clinton is our next president and I am very happy and hopeful about that. I wrote a letter for my friend Diego asking for early release. I hope it works, because he is another person who is in here for being under-represented. The legal system is just crazy and I want to do something to change that. I really think my depression is gone for good. I sure have God to thank for that. I have been restless today and not very optimistic about getting out. It is funny how it comes and goes. I sure want out and pray for it a lot. I am reading a book about a man who grew up in the Warsaw ghetto. There is some inspiration for perseverance.

November 5

I am feeling more at peace today. I almost got wrote up this morning for throwing food at someone who threw their food tray into the window. Apparently I hit C.O. Fortess and he was pissed. But thanks to God and because of a work ethic others talked him out of it on my behalf. Things like that really demonstrate to me the power of prayer. I was able to stay in touch with God, remain calm. Pray, and I did the right thing. I have gotten more insight tonight at Church. We know many of the things that please God. The Bible speaks of many of these and we just know many things that are good. We are never wrong for doing these and should always try to do them. But the idea is to do what God tells us, not what we think God tells us. This is a personal thing that is different for everyone. We must learn to trust that inner voice. We must realize that we cannot possibly understand all the ways that God works, but at the same time we must try. If I keep trying to live the right way I am happy. I learn through experience and this makes God and my beliefs personal to me. This is the process of growth. I really do think God has truly touched me, giving me knowledge, understanding, and joy. It is remarkable to me that me and Russ both had the idea of becoming full partners at the same time. I shall insist that we organize our money and set aside some for God. This will be a challenge with Russ, but when he sees how things go, he will be converted. I pray that these things will work out. I don't know how I am going to get out, but I still hope for the best. I was mistaken about the Judge being out of office at the beginning of the year. It is funny how beautiful people and the world are when I am in this light. I find myself being much less critical of things when I believe that everything is according to God. I always felt that these kind of thoughts were weakening; boy was I wrong. They are so paradoxical, though, that they are very hard to explain. I just know that I am going to keep moving forward. Things seem so much easier for me now. Discipline, although hard, just doesn't seem to be a nuisance anymore and it brings me satisfaction. I can not wait to get out, but the Lord makes this bearable.

November 6

The way peace of mind can leave me is boggling. It has been a rough day all around. I just wanted to curl up and escape from everything and let time pass. I am getting very tired of working in the kitchen, the laziness, the gaming, the bullshit. The blacks can really piss me off sometimes with their endless whining about their inferior treatment. Actually, no one usually messes with them because it's a waste of time to try to get them to do anything. They are always scheming and trying to pull something off on someone. I hate to talk that way about them because I like most of them very well, but it's the truth. I almost got in a fight with a stocky black named Quadem. We don't care for each other much, but have usually remained civil. Lately he has been trying to intimidate me because that's the kind of thug punk he is. Butch won't let him and it infuriates him. I will not let fear bully me nor will I be bullied. Screw him, he will be gone soon.

Roberto, who I told about the HIT program and wrote letters for was taken to work release today. I am happy for him, but a little frustrated that I have not gone over there. I do not understand. I went into Linda's office and explained and she called Joe for me. I guess it had something to do with qualifications. Joe said to be patient, that he was looking for a better job for me or something to that effect. I need to relax but I feel so discouraged lately about being here. I want out so bad and I am watching a lot of people leave; I can't wait for my turn.

Our Bible Study has let up lately and I am afraid I am with a band of jailhouse religionists. I talked to Ron about it tonight and he assured me that wasn't the case. He has had a lot of things happen to him lately and I thought he may have given up on God; I am more confident in him now.

I feel like withdrawing for awhile, like I need to let time pass. Mom talked to Dr. Ames and he thought it would be a bad idea to stop taking the Prozac right now. I think he is right, especially the way my moods have been gesticulating lately. I need to keep the faith and continue to grow. But I think I will give myself a little break and spend my time reading, writing, and exercising.

November 7

I had a much better day today. Corey was back on the dish line and we got the people working who are cool. We talked and joked around all day. Last night late, pat and I had a good talk about God. We discussed the personal nature of God. I still feel that he is a good works believer. That is a hard hurdle to cross and I now know the joy that Martin Luther felt when he had this revelation. I really know what people are talking about now when they say God found them. I was searching for happiness for so long and what I found was God. I really felt that teachings of Jesus are more like fatherly advice than commands, at least that is the way I feel about them.

We had a wonderful Church service tonight. It was one with pop music and a fired up preacher. The brotherhood and fellowship was tremendous. I have never seen so many joyful people in jail; the turnout was tremendous and the cornerstone Church people were overwhelmed and delighted. The preacher's message was exactly what I have been teaching. I asked God to let me know and he did in overwhelming fashion. I can't wait to put my faith into action outside of here. I want to live. I can't hardly believe I ever wanted to die. He talked about changing your heart, and changing your beliefs as the key to changing your life. It just blows me away how this has happened. I don't even know the magnitude of the change that has taken place, because I know I have not even consciously considered all of the changes in thinking that have occurred. I know that there are not gaps in my beliefs anymore and everything I believe makes sense, at some level.

November 8

Today was a good day also. I got along very well with everyone today and made it to Church this morning. With enough badgering, which I actually did in a very nice way, I have gotten the C.O.'s to come by the kitchen on Sunday mornings now for Church. We also had Bible Study tonight. We were pretty lax about it and I had some concerns about my fellows' sincerities. Pat did not show tonight and I am concerned about where his heart is. But, the big man came tonight. His name is Chuck. He is a huge black guy who I used to work with in the kitchen and who I play basketball with. I have always gotten along with him well, but I was surprised that he joined us. It was very refreshing and satisfying to have him join us. Going in there and having fellowship is always a nice respite from the day. I always leave feeling refreshed and happy.

I wrote Russ a long letter explaining some of my feelings today. I am very curious about his response but I feel it will be good because I think he has been thirsting for a change also. I also talked about things with Gary, the Pollock for a while tonight. We get along well and he is a smart fellow also. We talked about A.A. and things of spiritual ness also. It made me think about something. Because I feel that I drink because I am immature and have various problems doesn't give me an excuse to keep doing what I have been doing. It also means that just stopping drinking isn't going to fix them. I have to work at growing and achieving my goals. That is my salvation.

November 9

Today has gone well. It is my day off in the kitchen and what a day to have off. The dishwasher's heating element would not turn off yesterday when we were leaving. So it would not burn up, the second shift was not allowed to use it. (You really could use it as long as the coil was covered with water, but unfortunately the people who run the kitchen didn't take any chances.) Corey tried to use it this morning, but they stopped him and made them wash the dishes by hand while I napped. And people say there is no God.

I showered and shaved early today and read the paper. We went to rec, but I missed getting on a team right away and then things broke up because Chuck got hit in the eye. So I lifted weights. I am getting quite strong. I called Aubrey before work to see if he had found out anything; not a thing. I keep learning over and over that you have to take your life into your own hands. It's a lot more satisfying that way anyway. I'm going to call Richard tonight and see what's up and tell him that I expect him to do something. I am getting brave. I wrote Aunt Mary Ann and Uncle Bob today telling them how I'm doing and thanking them for writing.

I've got Monday Night Football coming up tonight as well as ACTS classes, so it should be a good evening. Tomorrow it's back to work and a Church service in the evening. I am trying to get out of the kitchen and found out how to do that today. In the process Linda, the case manager, said I would be going to HIT; but when?

So much for ACTS and Monday Night Football. The ACTS guy didn't show and because of our noise and one smart-ass, the C.O. turned off the game. Oh well, Bible Class went very well. I am really taking an active role in it. We read James Chapter one tonight; awesome. It has so many guides to good living in such a short space. Lines like "be quick to listen, slow to speak, and slow to anger," and "because he who doubts is like a wave of the sea, down and tossed by the wind." That was me, trying to live in two worlds. A man with no foundation, tossing from one thing to another. No wonder I didn't know right from wrong anymore. Now it is so simple, follow my heart.

I wrote three letters witnessing to the change that has taken place in me. That is something I never thought I would do. I am just so confident things are going to work out for me. I know I am on the right track.

Two people I like came to the dorm tonight. They are both relatively short timers, but it is always good to have friends. One is Rick Younger, who I used to work with at Tire man when he was still in high school and now lives down the street. The other is a guy from K-1 who I met and must say is serving the stupidest sentence I have ever heard about. He is serving 90 days on failure to appear for a charge that was dropped. He could get out anytime and for his sake I hope he does. He has been here 10 days longer than me.

November 10

Today was kind of a blaze' day. I started off the day in part of a racial incident which evolved from the way I was setting trays down. It was stupid, but I was ready to fight and threatened to tear the guys ass off. Eventually sanity came and I told the guy I was wrong and apologized. We got along well after that.

Bible Study wasn't too inspiring either. We read James 2, but none of us seemed too insightful. We ended up talking about anger, fighting, and people bugging us. I brought up praying for enemies idea and also about the idea that usually something else is bothering us besides what is obvious. I don't really have a strong feeling about praying for enemies so I am going to pray for understanding on that.

I talked to Richard tonight on the phone. My last letter was blunt and must have struck a nerve. He was not too impressed with it but he is filing my motion for early release. He doesn't have much hope that it will succeed, but as crowded as it is, who knows. I will pray about it and for Judge Blank. He said he will file another at 4 months. I will write to the judge before Christmas. Things are clicking.

Ron asked me to write his judge for him. I will do what I can; he has always been nice to me. He has a weapons charge on top of a record and I don't know what hope there is. I am trying desperately to get out of the kitchen but nothing has materialized yet. Another Maumee guy was released early so there is hope.

November 11

I have been pretty tired all day and spent the afternoon playing cards. Mom and Dad came for a visit tonight. We had a leisurely conversation about life, my plans and Susan and Rick. Jennifer really liked her first experience flying. I'll probably get to hear all about it on Saturday, if they make it out to visit. Susan and Rick already bought a house in Birmingham and sold theirs. Amazing Jennifer is very impressed with everything about moving.

Bible Study has not had the same punch for me and I don't know why. I guess before I felt like I wasn't learning so much and now it is a lot of reaffirmation. I think also I am getting to a juncture were I am not quite sure about a few things. I am starting to wonder about how literal to take things. I think I have to remember to take it easy.

November 12

Today went well. I began a new job in the kitchen cooking. I hated working on the line though and I needed a change. This is more independent work and that is better for me also. I am reading a book about Cicero. It is a novel by Taylor Caldwell and describes him growing up and the formation of his thoughts. It is very interesting and talks about getting in touch with yourself. I have decided that getting in touch with yourself and getting in touch with God is the same process. God gives you the courage and the reason to reflect on your life. He gives you the drive to search for truth and strive for greater things. Getting in touch with yourself gives you the confidence to know that who you are is good and unique, the courage to use your talents in the best way. It allows you to express in a variety of ways the truth and the beauty that you see. That sense of peace and joy overcomes any turmoil or suffering that is endured during the journey to those ends.

I received a letter from Beth today. She is very busy with Natalie. She said that she would enjoy a visit, but did not think that living with them was a good idea. It is ironic that I recently came to the same conclusion. I need to base my decision on where to live on more than on what is the most convenient. I think that was part of her reasoning also. I want to make my own way and have my own things anyway. I am tired of waiting, wanting and suffering. It is strange the way I was twisted, ever so slightly but completely out of synch. I always thought that my intelligence and abilities by themselves were enough to survive on. That by themselves I should be successful. Waiting for someone to discover my rare talents. Now it is as if this thought has been completely turned around. Everything I have is a gift. I can use these gifts to fulfill my dreams and aspirations. I simply have to decide what I want and go get it. God let me out to live. I think the thoughts that have been swirling around in my head are leading somewhere. My beliefs and convictions have miraculously changed. One of the biggest changes is not thinking of myself with respect to other people. I think this is the key to becoming selfless. And selfless is the key to living for yourself. Living for yourself is the key to finding God. And God is the key to happiness and fulfillment.

I always feel like sharing my ideas. Fulfillment is the key to happiness and God leads us to fulfillment. By getting in touch with ourselves, we discover what God has planned for us. We receive knowledge and wisdom, strength and courage. Some other beliefs that have changed are my ability to drink and smoke pot. The belief that these things shouldn't cause me problems is gone. Deluding yourself is dangerous. It severs your communications with your inner self and to God. The belief that my inclinations and natural feelings must be acted on because they are what I truly want to do. This is the doctrine of anti-discipline. Without discipline we can achieve nothing and therefore never be fulfilled.

November 14

It has been an eventful couple of days. Yesterday was Friday the 13th and it lived up to its billing. Work was hectic as I began my first day as the diet tray guy. Two people were written up: one for giving away a milk, and the guy teaching me the diet trays was removed for having a cigarette. That left me the job of preparing the trays and I had no idea what I was doing. Hale, the guy who was the cigarette smuggler, also produced a homemade wine, referred to as "hooch", in the kitchen. It was made of apples and had a strong taste, but wasn't really bad. I only drank one cup of it and got a little buzz. It made me kind of tired and I really never searched it out.

When I got back to the dorm I noticed a notice posted on Linda's door proclaiming that there were openings in the HITT program for people from Williams, Henry, etc. counties. I was again enraged about not being called. I waited for Linda and she never came. Finally after work she arrived and I asked her about it. Again she was vague, but told me that Joe Lane had asked about me and wanted to see me. He finally arrived about 5:00 and told me that he had a job for me. I am to work at a fertilizer plant. It is hard work and dirty. I told him I would do it. And he told me I would be moved on Saturday. At least it is steady work and I will get 40 hrs. a week.

Later that night I was told to pack up and that I was going to B-Dorm. This led to much speculation about me going home. That is usually the case and my friends in the dorm thought this. I knew it was too good to be true, but I hoped and dreamed.

I went into B-Dorm and ran into my old friend Roberto, who I had introduced to the HITT program. He has quit his job through the program and has been accepted to work in the shop of the construction company he works at. We talked for a long while and then I returned to my cell to read and sleep. Later that evening the C.O. called through the intercom to tell me I was moving to work release in the morning.

I called my Mother to tell her the news and asked her to buy me work boots and bring me clothes for work. I cancelled my visit, at Joe's Direction for today. She is bringing my stuff tomorrow. I was moved over to M-building, where the work release is housed, today about 11:00. It is pretty relaxed over here and I enjoyed my first coke in two months. Roberto loaned me the money. He offered, so I accepted .

God answers prayers. Now I hope he sees fit to release me from here. I will take what I get and thank him, for I am a lot better off than I was, even before I came into jail. I should be able to save quite a bit of money in here, I may end up staying the whole time. I hope I can stick out the job; I will just do what I can and not worry about it. I went to a meeting of alcoholics for Christ tonight. The leader is a born again and zealous Christian. I did not agree with him on everything, but those differences don't seem to matter to me anymore. I don't feel like I am competing, only sharing how I feel. It is very comfortable.

I found out that furloughs are a possibility for me. That is encouraging for I sure could use a break from here. They used to have a regular program for them out here but that has been suspended. Now you have to take it up with your Judge on your own. I will find out more about it when I have a meeting with Joe.

November 15

The cowboys lost today, but my fantasy team had a great day. I've been thinking hard again about how to get out of here. I prayed for wisdom last night. I do not think there is any way that the Judge is going to release me because it makes sense or it is the right thing to do. I was shocked to find out how many people from Maumee are here in the work release program. I don't know if the beds in here count the same for him as they do in the regular jail, but he has got a hell of a lot of people in Striker.

The book I am reading about the ancient Roman Cicero has made me think. His law teacher was talking about what motivates men and that law is a harlot, it goes to the one with the biggest purse. It has been making me wonder what motivates the Judge. I can not figure out a monetary motive. I guess the virtuous motive is possible, given the long standing mo- tive. I guess the virtuous motive is possible, given the long standing rumor about his daughter being killed by a drunk driver. But I still question this knowing that I went to school with his kids and never heard anything about it. If this is correct, maybe it is his record and reputation I need to at- tack. There have also been long standing rumors about his DUI activity. I have never been able to substantiate this and have been trying to think of a way. Well it came to me this morning. I remembered that a friend of Loretta's is a dispatcher for the County Sheriff and has access to driving records. I am going to call her tomorrow and see if she can get him to look up the Judge. If I can dig up some dirt on him and push the right buttons, maybe I can get somewhere.

This is kind of crazy, but I have also been looking at the computer system in the hallway here. I don't know if I can access Shamias, but I may try and see if I can adjust my out time. I'll have to make a serious plan before I try anything like that. I have just come to the conclusion that barring a miracle, which I pray for, conventional means are not going to get me out of here. I am still going to try, but I am going to concentrate on the unusual.

While I was writing, I was listening to some guys and joined in about this very subject. One, my Bunkie, said that his lawyer knows something about the Judge recently getting his 3rd DUI and that he is under some pressure from the city. We will see.

November 16

Slaves have nothing on me now. The man I work for should be ashamed of himself. I have to load 40 lb. bags of top soil onto pallets. I take them off a conveyor belt which pushes them out at 20 a minute. It's not so much that the job is hard, but the conditions suck. The day is atrocious, and it is incredibly boring. I just can't believe they don't switch things around. Standing in the same place throwing 40 lb. bags of dirt around for eight hours is a heck of a way to spend the day. It is better than sitting in jail, but just barely.

I wish I could think of a way to get a different job. I saw some decent jobs in the Blade again, but it just seems fairly impossible to get a job in my current situation. Maybe I could work with Russ; I don't know. I am thankful for the situation I am in and grateful to have a job, but this is going to be no piece of cake. I can endure. I have been trying to call Russ, but I can't get ahold of him. I need to write Beth back tomorrow, I'm going to watch Monday Night Football tonight if I can stay awake. The Proverbs of the day, "He who ignores discipline despises himself, but whoever heeds wisdom and humility comes before honor."

November 17

I was just talking to a guy who received 45 days from my Judge, who had a whole slew of charges against him. I just don't understand it. What the hell is Richard talking about. He was just about the biggest waste of $1000 ever and I plan on letting him know. I met one of the girls who works in the dirt factory today. She was actually pretty nice and looked just like you'd think, talked that way too. It has to be about the worst job ever, but I'm getting used to it. I am very tired and probably won't be up late tonight.

I got a response back from my case manager, dealing with the questions about the Judge. She did not give up much, but she gave me a lead. I talked to Russ about running the Judges' DMV report last night and that is in the works. That will be very interesting to see. I got a Thanksgiving card from Aunt Mary Ann and Uncle Bob. It's nice to know that I am in people's thoughts. I really can't get much done when I am working like this because I am too tired. I was going to write Beth and try and take care of some other things but forgot it.

November 18

Mom and Dad came out tonight. We had a very casual visit and I jokingly told them about my idea to invade Shamis. Mom is scared now. I really detest work and have got to change my attitude about it. I guess

I have just forgot how awful manual labor is, especially the minimum wage variety. I just find it hard to believe that people expect you to work your ass off for 4.25 an hour.

I wrote a couple of letters tonight. I wrote one to the Judge asking for a furlough or early release. I'm going to make him see Tim Niemann and suspended sentence as often as possible. I also wrote to the Lucas County Commissioner for information about my Judge. I sure hope that comes through for me. I am going to put all the facts to the people and see what they think about them. I'm hoping Russ comes through for me on that DMV report.

I am doing well with quitting smoking. It is bizarre how bad cigarettes smells to me now. Every once in a while I am tempted to smoke one, but for the most part, I can't imagine putting one of those stinky things in my mouth. It has been kind of a bad attitude day, but there were no confrontations and the day went pretty well. I'll pray for a better one tomorrow.

November 19

I feel healthy and full of life today. I had another computer lesson tonight. This one C.O. is very happy to display the functions of Shamis. It's going to take quite a move to use it, but I may think of something. We got out of work a little early today, much to my delight.

I have been thinking a lot about who I am. In this book about Cicero, I am reading, he displays a lot of the same characteristics and feelings I have. I am a good and righteous person; sometimes it is hard to live that way. To avoid being who you are, though, is devastating, more so to some than others. It seems that I am so intuitive anymore. Like when I ask God for something it magically occurs. I receive wisdom, tolerance, and relief from pain upon request. I am a person that must do what I feel is right. I cannot hide or avoid my feelings. They are always evident so I must have good and sensible intentions. I have learned that the only thing natural about men is that they are lazy, self centered, and afraid. You can pick the characteristics that you want, the ones you employ are your character. Character is not something you are stuck with, it is something you build. Your actions are primary, motives are slightly behind them, thoughts are way behind. This has been a revelation to me. What you do is all you have to worry about. If you do nothing, you feel like nothing. Its that simple.

November 21

Today has went well. I slept a lot after watching the OSU cs. UM game. It ended in a tie, first time I can remember that. I forgot to take my medication yesterday and I almost forgot to take it again today. I have been feeling a little disjointed and I wonder if that is it. I have been feeling alright, just not as spiritual as I have in the past.

I have been working out regularly and am getting pretty strong. I sure miss my Bible Study and Church that I was attending on the other side. I went to an Alcoholics for Christ meeting tonight. It was pretty nice. The guy in charge of it, Charlie, was a real down to earth person. I don't feel like writing much tonight.

November 22

I slept the day away again. I got up early and asked the C. O. to see if she could arrange for me to go to Church. It worked out and one of the Mexican guys I talk to, went with me. I talked to Pat over there and found out that after spending a couple of days in the hole, the charges were dismissed on him and he was reinstated into the trustee dorm. Ron is next door to me now in the county trustee program. We get to talk quite a bit now. My spirit seems to be coming back again. Church always seems to help focus me. That's what is important about fellowship. When we are on our own for too long, we start to wonder and get too wrapped up in ourselves.

I am finding that I have a lot in common with this Marcus Tullis Cicero, at least in thought. I am finding that the contemplation of philosophical ideals is also on the road to spiritualism. Seeking truth is seeking God, no matter how we go about it. It is impossible to keep things in perspective without having a good idea of who you are. You gain this perspective through meditation and prayer.

Through meditation, I can identify the affairs of my life that are bringing me trouble. Sexual relationships is one area I must begin to look at. I have been forcing it on the back burner for a very long time and I now realize that it is going to be a source of problems for me. My moral code is very complete, except in this area. I do not understand why adultery is a sin, yet I practice near abstinence because of fear of hurting someone. I know my thinking has been screwed up in this area. I still think about my love from high school constantly. Am I in love or just incredibly naïve and immature. I still dream about her. I miss that unconditional love and devotion. I guess I have not felt worthy of receiving it and have kept women at arm's length and would never let them feel that I thought they were important. Maybe this is another area of my life that will work itself out. I long to love again. I know I have to get my own life in order because my own feelings of inferiority have had an impact on my aloofness.

November 23

I am starting to feel optimistic about getting out again for some reason. I have continued to work out and am becoming a BMF. I have been praying a lot for wisdom on enjoying life. I tend to over analyze things and that will drive you crazy. It really takes the fun out of things. I have to learn the difference between things that come naturally and should be avoided and things that don't come naturally and should be sought. I am trying hard to become my own person. I want that person to be loose, cool and funny, but I am often stiff, serious and abrasive. I have to remember to take myself less seriously. I have been worrying about what I will do when I get out. About going right back to the way I was. This is kind of silly because I know I can do whatever I want when I leave. I know that there is nothing magical about pot or beer that is going to turn me into a monster. I just have to be careful and think about whether I want to use them at all anymore. I know for sure I don't want to use either one daily and that I would much rather abstain if that is the choice.

I guess I have just been caught up in pushing this Christian thing again. I have to remember the magic trick, to pursue slowly with open eyes and open mind, to let things come to me. This is such a complex idea because it is so simple. you must have some direction, but you don't have to have all the answers. The secret of life, the secret of finding God.

I have been thinking a lot about Florida again. I think that is where I would like to move or somewhere on the Ocean. I might have to check North Carolina out for school reasons. This Clinton thing might be just the ticket for me to go to law School. I am going to finish my degree as soon as possible.

November 24

Work wasn't too cool today. I stacked pallets all day and felt a little better about it. There were a couple of newcomers that did bullshit jobs all day. I am just a little resentful about us jail people getting stuck with all the hard jobs. I need to learn to take care of myself and not worry about everyone else. There is a nice way to do that without being deceiving and selfish. At the end of the day I kind of got into it with one of the guys out there. He is such a negative punk, he really bothers me. He came in to tell me to go clean up this huge mess outside. I told him no and went about my business. I have been trying to reach a point where I am willing to work and not feel too taken advantage of. I have to learn that I don't have to make everyone else agree with me to feel justified. This is a tragic flaw of mine.

I was talking to Dean, a friend of mine in here who I referred to on Sunday about Church, while I was writing. He came up kind of out of the blue and we had a discussion about our crazy lives. He lost his entire family in a car crash about 5 years ago and started drinking. He had 5 years of crazyness and is now trying to put his life back together. He thinks he just lost those 5 years. It is hard for me to look on my own life and say I lost 10. I know things would be different without the drugs and drinking, but I truly believe I am going to be a better man through all of this. A real man.

November 26

Thanksgiving day in jail was a somber day. I found my furlough denial stapled to the back of Chuck Schwin's furlough grant last evening. I was very disheartened and full of incomprehension. He was a man who has been to prison 3 times and has a driving record longer than War & Peace. He is 54 or so and making sort of a fresh start and is nice, but this is unbelievable. He also was granted one for Christmas. When my heart is broken like that I want to get out of here at all costs.

It seems as if I will never get out of here. I did not call anybody today nor do I plan to for awhile. I need to let some time pass and try to reconcile with God for a while. I am beginning to appreciate the duality of man and of the impossibility of certitude. We cannot even be certain of ourselves except at those rare times when we feel the serenity of God's presence.

I seem to have the pre-flu symptoms of an achy body, swollen throat and headache. I am not sure what I will feel like tomorrow, but it will be hard to go to work feeling like this. I have been very somber lately. Not that I have been hard to get along with (well a little), but I have just not sought the company of others. I have become aware at a deeper level of the lack of any "right" way to live. I mean there kind of is, but it lies in always reaching and working towards wisdom and knowledge. It requires discipline and sense of balance between work and play. A life devoted to happiness is found devotion to one's soul and his fellow man. A life devoted to pleasure leads to the death of soul, true misery. Pleasure is OK, but always dangerous and should be regarded as so. HAPPY - PLEASURE

November 27

There has never existed a wise man who did not know God. All great wisdom is divine inspiration just as all wise men have been touched by God. There is much to the world which is not known. This humility is the first step towards wisdom. It is foolish for a person to deride this religion or that belief, for all of us worship the creator. This spiritualism is the realization of our beings as a spirit and a belief in the Great Spirit. I believe there is a huge spiritual world that most of us know nothing about. To become attuned to it requires an open mind and a faith in that which we cannot see. I believe heaven and hell exist in this realm.

God's mercy for man is not understandable. He has given us the ability to be as He, but we are naturally drawn to immediate gratification and thus death. The suppression of this natural urge is the basis of spiritualism. It requires the love of and from the Almighty, which provides the power and inspiration to reach for greater things. Jesus came to reintroduce man to God and walk with him. They are a path to wisdom. The things we have on earth are gifts from God and not to be despised. We must remember that pleasure is only wrong when it becomes more important than God, which is easy to occur. Thus, pleasure is not to be despised either, but treated with care as a gift.

Since God has gifts for us all and a plan for each of us, it is important to remember the individuality of men, and not to be bogged down by the similarities of man. Although, we have much in common, just as it is wrong to believe we are better than someone, because they are different.

I have spent the day in that high attitude that always accompanies the flu in me. So I have spent much of the day meditating with the results of what I wrote before this. I did not go to work today and rested and read and thought. I hope I don't get any grief over it, but my body ached all over. The guys I worked with came home at noon because the machinery would not work with the wet and so we're not working tomorrow either. That's OK with me.

I have got half of the access code I need and have made further inroads on the computer. Now I need to make further plans to utilize them. I can get in the office this weekend and need to make the move if I am going to, I sure hate to mess up though. I have been talking with my neighbor about the Judge while I have been writing. What a strange character our Judge is. He hands out the strangest sentences. It seems that there has to be something someone can do about him. I will have to talk to Richard about it again.

I am starting to feel better physically as well as mentally after being down from this Thanksgiving thing. I am beginning to feel optimistic again. I know I can serve my whole sentence without losing my mind, but I sure want out. I am so anxious to live fo myself. No more waiting. Just the journey onward down the path of wisdom on the search for further enlightenment. It is funny to me that when some people find Christ it is the end of their search, for me it is the beginning.

November 29

Some of my despair has left me over the furlough deal, but my flu is still with me. I haven't exercised for 5 days now because of my fever. My mind has been muddled and I have not been at peace. I am having trouble remembering if I took my medicine. I am going to have to get in the habit of marking my calender. I went in the office today, but I was too chicken to try for the computer. I have spent most of the day reading, sleeping, and occasionally watching TV. I talked to my Mother and her soothing and compassionate voice was more refreshing than I imagined. She is going to get me a doctor's appointment.

I have been reverting to some of my perfectionist attributes. I sometimes slip into this visige that if you live a certain way, say the right prayers, have the right thoughts, things will magically work out and everything will be perfect. I know that there is a certain amount of truth to this but I can skew it into a frustrating plain of the obscure. Life is much simpler than this. I have to remember that I don't have to attain enlightened wisdom tomorrow. Just seeking and keeping in touch with God will be alright. You can't force life, even though I try awfully hard sometimes. Finding joy in the day as it comes is the way. My Christian yearning led me to be too hard on myself lately. Thus, I know things are askew a little bit. There are still some missing pieces to the moral pie. But maybe I am not supposed to have them all yet. I still have a lot of life to live. My goal is to lose some of my seriousness over the next few days. I have been very solitary and somber lately.

November 30

I hate my job. I forgot how much after this 5 day break. There are just some things I consider myself too good to put up with. I thought about this and was wondering if my heart was in the right place. I have to say that I must remember my situation, but I am way too good for that. I just have to keep plugging away and remember to just worry about what I am doing. Not what anyone else is doing. But the place and everyone in it drive me nuts.

I am going to the doctor with my Mom tomorrow and am really looking forward to it. A day off and time away from jail. I am looking forward to talking to the Dr. also. I want to find out more about this Prozac that I am taking. I was wondering also if I was being undisciplined about taking the day off when I don't really need to, give me a break. I take things so serious sometimes. That's what gets me into trouble. I make things so difficult. I feel obligated to throw the baby out with the bath water. It is hard to enjoy things like that unless you are perfect. I guess at one time I might have thought I was. Things are a lot simpler since I realized that I'm not and that I don't have to be.

I always wonder what I will be like when I'm free. I'm getting more and more confident that I will be grand. A couple of Allen boys got out today and that really cheered me up. Things are going to happen.

December 1

Ah, the beginning of another month. Two more boys from Maumee left today for a total of 7 so far. There is a rumor afloat that eight more are to follow and I can't help but to be filled with anticipation. I know better than to get my hopes up, but I can't help it. One of the guys who left today, rode the bus out here with me way back in September.

I went to see the Dr. today with my Mother. It was a grand time, almost like being friendly. We had a Pizza Hut pizza for supper. Went to see Susan and Jennifer. On coming back and telling my bunkee about my doctor, I come to find out that he sees Dr. Adas, amazing. The doctor was busy, but we talked a little and he gave me some antibiotics for my flu. Boy have I learned to appreciate the simple things of life. The doctor did think Prozac was helping me quite a bit. Be it the drug or God himself, it doesn't matter; I have found God, and happiness, and peace and drive. I feel anew. I feel full of compassion and full of wisdom. I am my own person. I have to prepare myself for the event that I don't get out. I am praying hard for it tonight.

December 3

I keep thinking I am getting rid of this cold, but in the morning I feel terrible. I worked yesterday and felt alright. We got today off for some reason, much to my chagrin. I have been quite the loner lately for some reason. I really don't have anyone in the work release facility that I get along with especially well. Not that I have been so disagreeable to others, just no closeness. Maybe it's because I am so excitedly anticipatin my early release. Another case of the short syndrome (everyone turns into a cocky dick when they are about ready to get out of jail) One of the pain in the ass VOA'S (Victim of Allens) talked to his attorney the other day and said that he is going to court Friday. He has about the same time served as I and told me I would be going with him. I hope he knows something I don't, because I really want to go.

I have not felt oh so serene the last couple of days. Maybe I can't expect to feel that way all the time. The worries of the world creep into my thoughts without regards to an invitation. I am still feeling pretty darn good mentally though. I can't even imagine considering suicide anymore. That Prozac must do something, but I am also sure of my God and spiritual being. I have come to understand the faith of children and the ignorance is bliss phenomenon as a conscious understanding that it is not necessary to understand everything at a conscious level. Everything makes sense, but not necessarily through reason or logic. Some things just feel right, even though they cognitively have no place, operating to ones full potential. The spiritual side of one's life is an important and powerful thing.

I have been trying to decide how to use the day. I have put a lot of things off since I have been sick and have been anticipating my release. I haven't been physically active for awhile, even though I did push up last night. That routine of physical exercise and meditation is one I do not want to get out of. I am up to almost 200 pounds now and it feels great. I would like to start running 3 or 4 miles in the morning and do my push ups and sit ups. That way I should lose my new gut and continue to build legs and chest and maintain my weight. I am going to have to get used to cooking again. I'm going to need money. I am sure God will provide.

I guess I will do laundry today, organize my belongings and read. I just don't feel good about exercising yet. I still feel sick. I should write Aunt Betty and Uncle John maybe. I hope I can do a lot of visiting soon. I am so tired of that bizarre self-centered life I was leading. I as always either too ashamed or too selfish to let anyone into my life. Both aspects have seemingly disappeared along with the weight of the world. Before I always compared myself with everyone, and I mean some ridiculously successful people, and wondered why I could not match them. I expected to be a virtuoso at everything or I did not want to be anything. Now, I just want to use my gifts however I may and try to reach my highest aspirations, without much regard to what the world thinks. I think it is going to be a lot more satisfying this way.

December 4

I didn't make it out again, but Chuck Schutz did and he has quite a record. He had more time in than I, but I still thought I would beat him out. He said there was a stack of papers to go through, but he is not the most reliable of sources. I still have a lot of hope that I will be released soon. Hopefully sometime next week, cause I can hardly stand to work much longer.

Today we were asked to work tomorrow, which is Saturday. I said no, because I had a visit planned for tomorrow afternoon with Russ and Rachael. It did not seem a problem, but upon arrival Joe had me come into his office and asked me how I was feeling. I told him I was feeling much better. He then wanted to know why I wasn't working tomorrow, almost insinuating that I was up to something. I explained, but it was to no avail, I have to work tomorrow. It really pisses me off, but what the hell. I can endure being a slave for a while longer. I can just terrorize Brad, that's good for entertainment.

He wouldn't let me reschedule my visit either, which I think really sucks too. Hopefully I will be out soon and it won't matter. With the shock of Schutz getting out tonight, I had another lesson in trusting God. I get so apprehensive sometimes. I just have to remember that the things that are out of my hands are in His hands, and that the things in my hands are gifts. This idea is very reassuring and is assuming new meanings for me.

December 5

My forced labor went fairly well today. We did not run the line very much today and spent most of the day doing odd jobs around the place. My disenfranchise with my coworkers is continuing. In this mild altercation with Danny today. I found out he resents the way I work. Maybe my negative comments about the place and work in general rubs him the wrong way. I just don't have much in common with that group, but I should still be smart enough to fit in and not flap my mouth. I will try to be more positive, but I just don't understand why he would care what I do. I don't know if he is jealous of my laissez-faire attitude, or if I am way out here. I am just trying to make the place bearable. Working my butt off is not bearable.

I napped for awhile when I got home and now it is 1 A.M. and I can't get to sleep. My "cold" is showing no signs of subsiding. I almost feel real bad, but in the morning I feel awful sometimes. I'm almost wondering about pneumonia. God seems to be granting wisdom again today. I feel that His coming to earth as Jesus was to show us how to find Him and to remove guilt from our lives. That is the taking away of sins. The Trinity is still a hard concept for me and I still kind of think of the Godhead as three separate entities. But, perhaps that is the way it is.

I am optimistic about getting released soon, but have realized I needn't concern myself with it. I need to get out of myself a little and care for my fellows. There are many here in much tougher circumstances than I. God has not forsaken me.

December 6

I went to Church twice today! I was allowed to go over to the main building this morning where I got to see some of my old friends. When I returned I found out that my prayers and effort had been rewarded and we were going to have a service here in work release. The theme of both services was that Jesus changes lives. If we ask for something believing he will give it, he will. I keep hearing of experiences almost like mine where it seems as if Jesus found me. I have not been giving Jesus due credit, I think lately, for leading me to God the Father. It still is a kind of a confusing relationship to me, but it is clearing up. I had some excellent Christian fellowship today. I feel like I am maturing quickly. I realize now that I don't have to give in to my whims and thoughts; actions make the man. I am also realizing that balance is the key to life. Pleasure, pain, happiness, and sorrow, joy and boredom are all part of life. There is no way around it in the maturing cycle of purification through fire.

I have thought about my problems with my coworkers. I need to humble myself a little bit and make sure I am not belittling them. I don't think I need to worry about it too much, but I do want to show concern. I need to learn to be a little more political. I am trying not to worry about when I get out and just trust God to handle it for me. I feel more at ease and am continuing to pray on the matter. I looked in the classifieds and saw quite a few interesting jobs to apply for.

December 7

I almost went to bed without writing. I have been preaching my message of self discipline so I felt obligated to get up and write a little bit, for this has been great therapy for me and I do not want to lose this habit. Two more people are going to court tomorrow. I am happy for them, but I sure wish I was going too. I do not feel distressed though because I really do trust God. I feel sure that I will be out soon. He was maybe going to talk to the judge tomorrow. I would just like to know if the judge has some hard on for me.

I was not awoken by the C.O. this morning and my fine coworkers neglected to do anything about it. I awoke at 7:30 as they were heading out the door. I was kind of pissed for awhile but I did not lose my cool at all. I informed the C.O. and Joe Lynde as soon as possible. Joe ended up taking me to work at 9. We only worked a half day and I refrained from getting nasty with anyone. Tomorrow should be an easy day and hopefully my last.

I was talking to one of the guys who is leaving tomorrow about God and life a little tonight. I can talk so openly with the right people anymore. He was reading "The Road Less Traveled," and I talked to him about that. About how it helped me realize that we need not be controlled by our whims and desires. How self control and discipline are tools we can use to overcome our natural tendencies of laziness and direct us onto the road to success.

This is where Tim's journal ended. I assume he was released at this time.

5

Diagnosis: Bipolar Disorder

In Tim's journal of October 27 he mentioned writing a letter for a Puerto Rican guy, who didn't write English well. At times, Tim would call me from jail and ask me to call the parents of another young man in jail to let them know where their son was. Tim would also give me the young mans mailing address to give to his parents. I would always call the parents but I never knew what I would be getting myself into. I remember one time, while he was in jail in Florida, Tim asked me to call a mother in Ohio and tell her where her son was. The young man and a friend had left Ohio to seek employment in Florida, but hadn't been successful. I don't remember what he had done to be in jail, but he was also bipolar. She was very nice and we discussed our sons and their disorder for some time on the phone.

When Susan or I would tell Tim how we felt about him, how his drinking and irresponsible behavior was upsetting all of us, he would look so pathetic and sad. He never argued with us, he would agree and say he was sorry. He always said he would try to stop.

In fall of 1990 I went to a bar after work with co-workers. On way home a cruiser started following and that was it. Sentenced to 6 months and was released after 2 ☐ months.

The next year Tim entered a thirty-day inpatient substance abuse program in a local hospital. He stayed sober for a few months. Then in May of `91 he was living with a high school friend and his girlfriend. Tim called one day almost in tears. He said he had had a headache for a week and had taken everything he could think of, but nothing had helped. I asked him if he would go to my doctor, and Tim said he would. Then he said, "Mom don't worry, I am not going to do anything". My fear was a brain tumor. Paul's brother died from a brain tumor at age thirty-one. I picked Tim up and took him to see my doctor that afternoon. The doctor and I had talked several times about Tim and his alcohol problems, so this visit wasn't too much of a surprise. The doctor talked to both Tim and I, and assured me that there wasn't any need to worry about a brain tumor. He prescribed some medication he thought would help him, with the promise from Tim that he would return if he didn't feel better.

After a particular depressing period, when I was unpredictable and scary, a friend suggested that there was probably something that could be done for me. The thought had never occurred to me. I saw my parents doctor and he prescribed Prozac and introduced me to the world of psychiatric drugs.

At some point during this time, Susan offered to let Tim live with her family. I tried to talk her out of it, because she had a toddler to take care of and she didn't need to worry with him. It wasn't long before she told him to leave. He went to live with Russ again, his high school friend.

In May '92, while we were out of town, he came to our house, found the keys to our car, took it out, got drunk, and got another DUI. After his jail time, I received a call from Russ. He and his girl friend could not take Tim living with them anymore. He didn't want Tim to be on the street, so would I please let him live with us again? I told him no, and that he wasn't really helping Tim by letting him stay there either. I told him that Tim needed to wake up and realize what he was doing. Russ had told Tim to leave, but he hadn't left. I told Russ he should do as I had done one time, and leave all Tim's things in a garbage bag on the porch. Then Tim would leave. The next day Tim was at our door. I told him we wouldn't let him live with us, and told him he should ask our Pastor if he knew of a place that might take him in. He made an appointment to see the pastor the next day, and spent the night with us. Pastor was able to get him into the Salvation Army ninety-day program. On some Sundays we would go to Church with him there. It was a wonderful program, and it helped him find a good job.

Completed the 90 day program, obtained a job as a programmer, and rented an affordable house. Was well established, but after about 6 months, I began drinking and then even crazier activity. Held job for 2 ☐ years.

Tim was hired as a programmer at an office in downtown Toledo. After possibly six months, Tim seemed to be having some problems again. During this time, he had written a program and when he looked at it weeks later, he said there was no way it could possibly be done. After he was diagnosed bi-polar, we learned that he had been in a manic phase at that time. His program was more of a dream than reality. Also during a manic phase he felt he was capable of doing anything he wanted and never being punished for it. He did not like the manic phase at all. That is usually when he got into trouble.

As my life improved, I was still having occasional flair ups and was sometimes depressed and suicidal. My parents doctor agreed to continue prescribing as long as I saw a Psychologist. After doing this for a year and a half, she diagnosed me with manic-depression and referred me to a Psychiatrist. She also said for Mom and I go to the library and read everything we could find on Bipolar Disorder.

Tim moved back in with us again. He said he was glad there was a name for what was wrong with him, because he had thought he was just plain crazy. We did read everything we could find. One of the first things Tim discovered was that some of the great artists and musicians were suspected of being bipolar. The information, was a little scary, and I felt so bad for Tim having to be saddled with his condition. It was said to be hereditary, but we didn't know of anyone else in the family diagnosed with it. Tim said he could think of a few good possibilities. My sister said our maternal grandmother's sister, - which would be Tim's great-great-aunt, was mentally ill and lived some of her life in an institution. Mary Ann said she could remember going to Grandmothers and seeing our aunt laying on the couch, never speaking. We wondered if perhaps she might have been bipolar.

6

Colorado

1995 I was placed in the hospital by the Psychiatrist for adjusting and experimenting with the meds. I was fired from my programmer position, due to my inability to think, remember and function. Decision was after less than two weeks since release from hospital. I felt wronged. Later that same month, I entered another mental health treatment & meds.

After securing a programmer job in Denver, Colorado, I was very excited and felt that my life was going to take off. I had spent 3 weeks in the psych ward getting medication and had been sober for a few months. I had bought a car and had accumulated about $4000 for the trip and getting an apartment.

He never saved any money! When Tim wrote this, he must not have been doing well. Paul had given him $2500 in traveler's checks so he could get to Denver and find an apartment. I was against giving him so much at one time. I wanted to give him just enough for food, gas, and a motel, then take care of the apartment when he found one. One of the characteristics of bipolar disorder is that suffers cannot take care of their money. They often buy ridiculous things.

The first thing I did was buy a twelve pack of Miller and an ounce of smoke and I was on my way. It took until evening to reach Davenport, Iowa and the Casinos. It took another 3 days to lose all my money. I did not know what to do. I could not think of going back to Toledo. I continued to Denver, not knowing how this was going to work out. I just stole everything I needed, gas, beer, food. Somehow I made it and started working. I dined and dashed at Perkins. Police were in restaurant. A woman Sergeant caught me and she could see there was something wrong with me. She took me to detox and allowed me to go after I talked with psychiatric. Sentenced to weekend course on stealing.

Tim was to call us when he arrived in Denver, but we never heard anything. I finally went to the police and they put him on the missing persons list. The next day he called, a rather sad, panicking individual. We were angry, but helped him again. We called a motel and paid for a week's stay. We also sent him a little money, and that was going to be all. We told him this was his last chance. He had such a well paying job, in an area where he had always wanted to live. We had camped in Colorado many times: it was our favorite place. We prayed that he would straighten out and take care of his illness.

He seemed to be doing alright and he asked us if we might come out in the summer and bring Jennifer, our granddaughter. We decided to do that and he was so excited. He had an apartment by then and was having fun buying furniture, pictures, and so on, to make it look like home. We arrived before he was able to get home from work, and the manager let us in. Jenny and I looked over the apartment. It looked very nice. We even looked into the kitchen cabinets. Everything was clean and in order. He had a lot of plants in his living room. The furniture was nice and there were framed pictures on the wall. We hadn't known what to expect, but we were very happy with what we found - with Tim. One day he took us to his office to meet his boss. Another day we went sightseeing to places that Tim thought Jennifer would like to see: a butterfly exhibit, the mall at Boulder, Mesa Verde Indian Village, and the Rocky Mountain National Park.

We left for Maumee, Ohio on Monday, feeling hopeful that Tim would be able to stay sober and lead a decent life. But it wasn't to be. He began to get into trouble again. He lost that job but quickly found another programming position. I wasn't able to reach Tim by phone for a few days, so I called his office and talked to his boss. He told me Tim had received a traffic ticket and was taking care of it. I asked him why he had hired Tim, knowing he had bipolar disorder and the problems that went with it. He said, that Tim was the best programmer they had ever had and that they all liked him and wanted to help him.

7

Michigan

Tim stayed in Colorado for several years. He lost his job and started living with a girl who also had some mental issues. They got into an argument, which escalated into her calling the police, saying Tim had hit her. He was at his lowest, at this time. Here we were again: Tim came to live with us and get himself straightened out. Soon he had a programming position with a large company in Michigan, so away he went to try again to be on his own.

Paul had just retired and we rented a place in Winter Haven, Florida, for two months. While in Florida, I called Tim's apartment and received no answer, so I called his desk at work and left a message. He didn't call me back. The next day I called his boss, who told me that Tim had called one morning and said he felt bad and was going to the doctor, and they hadn't heard from him since. The man said he would stop by Tim's apartment and see how he was. I called Tim's answering machine again and left a message that I had left many times before: "Tim, if you don't answer, I am going to call the police." He immediately picked up the phone. He was so sad. He said he felt horrible and hadn't been able to get himself to work. He said he needed to see a psychiatrist. I told him I would catch a flight home and get him to one. The next day I went to Michigan, not knowing what I would find.

Several times, I had gone through this type experience with Tim, and each time I would be expecting to find him dead. Then I would be so relieved to find him alive, but oh, so sad. When he was in these phases, when he couldn't get himself to work, I would find him sitting on the floor, the room as dark as it could be, and him looking like the devil. He wouldn't have washed, shaved, or eaten anything. These were times when I had no one to talk to. Who would understand what was going on? My sisters thought that if he would only quit drinking, he would be fine. He told me later on, that bipolar people drink because they feel better drunk, than experiencing what goes on in their mind sober.

When I arrived at his apartment, Tim looked so pitiful. He cried and we talked. The next day we went to his psychiatrist and she placed him in a hospital for a week. When he got out he had a court appearance for a DUI. He was sentenced to jail for six months. So I called his boss, and he stopped over to pick up some things had that belonged to the company, and we had a nice talk. I then called Tim's friends, Russ and Rachael, to see if they could come up from Maumee. I would rent a truck if Russ would drive Tim's belongings back to our house in Maumee. I terminated the apartment rental, and Russ, Rachael, and I packed up Tim's belongings and took them to my house. I then flew back down to Winter Haven.

Before Paul and I left Florida, we bought a manufactured home in an over fifties park. So we were now having to make a lot of decisions. the girls and their families came up to spend the last Christmas at our home in Maumee. We went all out on the decorations and it was a great holiday.

Paul and I decided we wanted to do something special for the families. Our sons-in-law and the grandchildren had never been to Disney World. So we asked them all to get time off work the first week in June of the next year and we would take them all to Disney. I went to AAA to make the arrangements. I didn't make a reservation for Tim, since we wouldn't know if he was going until the last minute. In the end, he did go with us. Paul and I had a conversion van at that time and we all met at Susan's home, near Atlanta. Beth Anne and her husband drove down from Memphis in a rented van. We decided that all the girls would go in my van and all the fellows would go in Beth's. We were so happy to go on that trip. It was so much fun, since the kids and their fathers had never seen anything like Disney World. It was our first and last trip all together.

Tim would plan out each day, so the grandchildren would get to see and do their thing. He loved those three girls. On our last day we went to Daytona Beach and the girls rented bikes and played in the ocean.

In August of that year, I had my knee replaced. I wasn't to go up the stairs yet, so I slept on the living room couch and Tim said he would sleep on the family room couch. He said that way if I needed help he would hear me. The couch was low, so I needed help getting up and Tim was strong. He would help me do the exercises and walk with me up and down the sidewalk. He could be such a loving kind person and so much fun. I asked God so many times why does he have to have this disorder. But I knew God had his reasons, we just had to go on with our lives.

Tim and I were so close. He and I were a lot alike. We both liked nature, antiques, art, learning, exploring new areas, and people. We were alike too, in that we both kept sayings we liked in a file. I didn't know he did, till going through his files after his death. I don't believe he knew I did.

8

Florida

The last day of October, Paul, Tim, and I moved down to Florida. We were hoping Tim would find a job and move out on his own. Tim was fine for a while, but he needed to get out of the community where we live. He started going to AA and he met a nice young man to hang out with. His sponsor would have get - togethers at his home for them. Tim bought a scooter, so I wouldn't have to take him around all the time. His friend from AA would pick him up to go places. After several years had gone by, Tim became very down and suicidal and stopped by his sponsor's house, hoping to get some words of wisdom. Tim told him he felt like giving up and ending his life. Instead of importing wisdom, the sponsor told him, "we all have to go sometime". Well, that really sit him off. He was so angry and depressed. Since Tim didn't want me to worry anymore than I already did, he did not tell us any of this for quite some time.

He was getting very down, didn't have much to say, was doing a lot of thinking. One day he said he wanted to go into the Detox in Bartow, Florida. He had been there before and we were able to get him in again. After several months, he went into a half way house in Southern Florida. He wasn't there too long and he was asked to leave. The reason being, that he had moved the bedroom furniture around to suit him better and then he had words with someone in charge. Someone from AA let him move in with him and he started working in construction for another fellow from AA. Tim would ride his scooter over to the fellow's house and give him a ride to work. This went on for some time, and the man started mentioning he was having money problems. One day Tim arrived at his house and found him dead. He had committed suicide. This of course threw Tim into a depression. He called and we talked and he was so down. I asked him if he wanted to come back with us for a while, which he did.

The first evening he was back with us Tim asked if he could use the golf cart and go down to visit a friend who lived near the front gate. I couldn't go to bed for worrying about him. It was getting late, so I got into our car and went past the friend's house. No golf cart or Tim. I saw our golf cart parked by the front gate, parked out of the way. I drove out of the park and down the road looking for our son, but I didn't find him so I went home and told Paul and we drove down to get the golf cart. An hour later Tim came walking in and asked why we had taken the golf cart. I told him we were concerned about him. Paul went to bed and Tim and I sat in the screened porch, just off the living room, talking. That is when he told me about his talk with his AA sponsor about how he felt, and the sponsor's answer. We talked into the wee hours of the morning. He also told me he had contemplated stepping out in front of a semi-truck, while he was out walking that night, but that he finally couldn't do it. He and I both had tears. He said he wanted to go to an AA meeting in the morning and then see his psychologist and get some help.

The next morning I took him to an AA meeting and he said he would get a ride home. He never came home that day. He ended up walking to his sponsor's house. In the late afternoon, I received a phone call from the sponsor. His wife had seen Tim riding away from their home on the sponsor's bike. I told him I would have Tim call when he got home. So I decided I would try to find Tim. I drove around places where I thought he might be, but I could not find him. Later that night, the sponsor called to say that Tim was in jail. the police and that they had Tim and he was in jail. The next morning Tim's friend from AA called me and we talked. He told me how to get on the internet and find out which jail Tim was in. When I found it, I almost fainted. Tim looked terrible in the picture, and I saw a red line around his neck. The charges were Burglary of structure, grand theft, battery on law enforcement officer. I was horrified. Tim had never been violent before. I immediately went to the police station and asked an officer where my son was and if he had hung himself, because I had seen a red line around his neck. I also wanted to know how badly the officers were hurt. He pulled out the reports. He told me that, yes, Tim had hung himself in the cell with his boot strings, and when the officers saw him they rushed in and cut him down. He told me not to worry about the officers; one had hurt her pinky finger, and that charge would be dropped. I felt a little better; I hated to think that he had hurt someone. The week he died, he was to go to court to try to have the charges dropped.

When Tim was in jail for this offense, he had a public defender, as he usually had. This one did not seem to like Tim, and I can't say I blame him, in a way, but he was there to defend Tim. Two different mental professionals had called me and said Timothy needed to be placed in a hospital, he was in such a mental state. They asked me to tell the public defender to subpoena them so they could go before the judge and tell him Tim needs help. I told the public defender, but he did nothing. In court, Tim's mental issues were never mentioned.

Tim told me he had been in the depths of hell and he didn't want to go there again. He said he was seeing little tiny scary people and they were yelling things to him. He did not want to go through that again. Tim wrote a letter of complaint and the judge appointed a lawyer to handle the case and it was scheduled to be dismissed the week of the accident.

After Tim had served his time for that offense, Paul and I purchased some land that had two trailers on it. The double-wide one for Tim, and we thought he could rent out the second one and have some income to live on. The land was just under an acre and fenced, and there were chickens to take care of and a lot of fruit trees and tropical plants. There also was a mallard duck living with the chickens. The property was in a poor area, but we didn't think about it being a drug and theft area. For the first six months or so, Tim did fine. I worked with him a lot on fixing up the yard and the single-wide trailer. He researched how to clip the chickens' wings so they wouldn't fly out of the pen. He would catch them and hold them and I would clip them. He named a few of them. There was a chubby hen that loved to get out of the pen. We kept the chicken feed in a trash can and as soon as she would hear the trash can open, she would come a- running to get fed. She never missed a meal. Tim named her Miss Purdy.

There was also a little stream running through part of the property. The chickens thrived and before long there were baby chicks all over the place. Mr. Waddlesworth, the duck, seemed to think he was a chicken. Tim was determined to teach him he was a duck. One day Tim caught the duck and put him into the stream. He looked so happy swimming around, but all of a sudden he heard a chicken cluck and he took off flying right back to the chicken yard.

Tim was getting lonesome and bored, and he started visiting with the neighbors. Well, it became his downfall. He started getting into difficulties. Whenever I knew of a problem, I didn't hesitate to call the sheriff's office. I got to know some of the deputies, for the same ones often came out. I told Tim one day, "I bet when your neighbors see my car coming, they say 'Oh, here comes the bitch again.'"

"No, Mom, they like you and respect you, but you scare the hell out of them," he replied. I told an officer that I didn't know why they would be afraid of me, an old lady. He said, "It's because you will call us."

In September of 2005, Tim was in such a state that I asked my doctor if he knew of any place I could get Tim some help. Tim had no insurance or money. The doctor said to take him to the emergency ward at the local hospital, where they would have to admit him. Tim and I went, and we both were interviewed for some time. At the end, the person said Tim had a good doctor at the clinic he had been going to, and to make an appointment with him. I took Tim home and he called for an appointment and told the receptionist he was in a bad state of mind. The first appointment they could give him was in January, the same week of his accident.

9

Tim's Last Days

Tim, finally got tired of living in the trailer. He told me we should sell it and find something in a better area. I think he had fallen in with some of the drug people too deep and was afraid. I went over one day and there was a van by his trailer. I said, "do you have company"? He told me yes, that Mark had walked down to the store. A few days later I stopped by and the van was still there. Tim gave me another reason why the fellow wasn't there. He knew I was getting suspicious. I knew Tim well enough to know he was up to something. I was afraid that he was going to do something so that the deputies would have to shoot him, or was going to try to kill himself in an accident. I did not want anyone else to get hurt. That weekend, I told Paul, "I am going over Monday morning when I wake up and call the Sheriff if the van is still there and see if it is stolen. Paul didn't look happy about it. But come Monday morning I went over and it was there. A deputy came and ran the license number; it was stolen. He called for back up. I told the officers exactly where Tim would be and gave them a key to the trailer. One of them said, "Thank you Mom." I said, "This isn't fun for me, but I don't want anyone else to get hurt". Well, in they went. One of them came out to me and said they had him and he wasn't talking. I said he would talk when he saw me out side and knew it was me who had called. He went in, and the first deputy came out and said he would move his car so I could leave and Tim wouldn't know. So I left.

When I got home, Paul said, "Don't you know what you have done to him?" I said, "I didn't do it, he did it." We went over later to make sure the trailer was locked, and to our surprise Tim was there. After we left I called the deputy in charge, and he said they didn't have enough evidence to charge Tim. They had towed the van and taken fingerprints. It would take some time to run the prints. Well, the next evening my son-in-law in Georgia received a call from Tim. He told him he was close to their house, but couldn't remember how to get there. He followed their directions and arrived at their house. My daughter, Susan, and her husband knew what had happened the day before. Susan said he looked horrible and asked him whose car he had. He told her it belonged to a friend of his who was in jail and he had told him he could use it. They sat down and talked. He said that where he had been living was hell, and he couldn't stand it anymore. He wanted to go back to Colorado. Susan and Rick tried to reason with him: he didn't have any money - how did he think he could get there? They fixed supper and talked some more. Susan and Rick finally talked Tim into going back down to Winter Haven so he wouldn't worry Mom and Dad to death. Rick said he would fill the car's tank if Tim would then go home. . Tim said he would. He was worn out, and he went up to take a shower and go to bed.

When Susan thought it was safe, she went out and checked the car and found a car seat in the back seat and clothes with price tags on them. So he had been stealing things all the way, including the gas. She found a girl's billfold and took in the house with her. She then called and told me what was going on.

A detective from the Winter Haven police had already taken a report from me; I called and told him the car make and license number and the name in the billfold Every time that Tim had been in trouble before, it was for drinking or drugs, and here in one week he had stolen two cars. To everyone's surprise, he returned home. But the second day home, he drove at high speed into a light pole and the car rolled and he ended up with a broken neck and paralyzed from the neck down. He was flown to the hospital and lived four days. When Paul and I went to see him in the hospital, the first thing he said was, "Mom, I'm not going to make it." I tried to tell him he was young and strong and would be alright. He thanked us for coming. He was in so much pain, they put him into an induced coma. One by one his organs started shutting down. When he died, we left the hospital and called our daughters. Our granddaughter Jennifer, who was close with Tim, when she was told, she ran upstairs crying. Fifteen minutes later, she came down and handed her mother a paper on which she had written her thoughts of Tim. It was Jennifer's eighteenth birthday. Susan told me it was beautiful, and she thought Jennifer should read it at the funeral. The pastor agreed.

Jennifer read her paper at the service, but it was hard, for tears were flowing. Tim had once said to me, "Mom, please help Jennifer, she is so much like me. I am afraid she is bipolar." I told him there wouldn't be anything I could do. She is a lot like her Uncle Tim, but I think, she has just his good traits. She writes beautifully, she is very intelligent, and she likes people, especially the elderly. The following is what she wrote upon hearing of Tim's death.

Uncle Tim

Pretty much everyone knows that when I was a young girl, I idolized my Uncle Tim. I adored him. I know that he was not perfect, but I also know that no one ever is. Yes, when I was little, I was naïve, and I didn't know or understand everything. But I am glad for that. When you are a kid, it seems that you always see the positive in people, and not the negative. What a blessing that is!

The world is so new, and there is no room in your heart to think of the negative things in life. The heart of a little kid is so forgiving. And I like it that way. When I was little, my Uncle Tim was my everything. I looked at him as the most beautiful person. He was incredibly smart, he was funny, and he was so much fun. That's how I want to everyone to think of him. I want everyone to think of him through the eyes and the forgiving heart of a child.

Jennifer Anne

Jennifer wrote the following poem about a month after Tim's death.

Uncle Tim

I know you are in a better place,

But the thought of your absence is something I can't face.

I know one day I'll see you again.

But how do I get by until then?

There's so much more I want to say to you,

Like how my faith in you was genuine and true.

Towards the end I had nothing to say

But please know my love for you never went away.

One day I want you to look down on me

From your heavenly cloud.

And realize that I have made you very proud.

You will be in my heart until we meet again.

I know I will see that beautiful grin.

I love you, Uncle Tim

One day, in a self help group in Florida, Tim had to write a list of friends that he could depend on for help. He was able to list three. Beau, his friend from AA; Kathy, a daughter of our friends in Florida; and Russ, his friend from high school. What is so terrific about these three is that all were in attendance at Tim's memorial service. Tim knew who was dependable.

Another of his friends from high school, Dave, sent us the most beautiful letter after Tim's death. Dave said Tim was his best friend all through high school and college. Dave felt bad that he had not kept up with calling or writing Tim. When I answered his letter, I told him it was not his fault. Tim was embarrassed that he hadn't been able to go on with his life and own things like his friends, so he stayed away from them. Dave also thanked us for including him in with our family. He said he had always felt welcome, and he was embarrassed for not telling us sooner. He also asked us to tell the girls how much they had meant to him. His other really good friend, Dave from Des Plaines, Illinois, was so upset when he heard about Tim's death. The two of them were as close as brothers could be. Months later he called to talk to us, but when he heard my voice, he started sobbing. He has had a hard time accepting that Tim is gone. It also hit the cousins hard, for Tim was the youngest one. I think it made all the younger people realize how precious life is and how soon it can be over. It has made many of the younger generation look at what they are doing and to make their life more meaningful.

10

Tim's Business Dream

I am going to trust my creative instinct in the pursuit of my lifes calling. I figured this out quite a while ago. But I was still burdened with a lot of baggage holding in old patterns and thinking. My lifes calling is not some grand scheme or earth shattering ventures. And even if it is, I only accomplish it day by day and bit by bit. The only guides I have are my collective knowledge, my spiritual and moral understanding, and most importantly, my likes and interests. The things that make me feel good. I say this is most important because it encompasses everything else. It is the reliable compass that factors in the myriad influences that synthesis that incredible feeling when we are occupied with our work; with God's work.

My work involves history, and people, and what makes them the way they are. This found by experiencing what they experience. Eating what they eat, participating in their leisure activities, being with the art, dressing as they, learning their religion. To be involved in the cultures of the World, past and present, would be the experience of my lifetime. Bringing my dream and knowledge to others is how I plan to support myself.

To this end, I plan on bringing my culture and interests to others in dynamic store setting. I plan on being a trader in the grand tradition of making exciting goods available at modest prices in a fun and leisure setting. A place where one could enjoy a variety of coffee and other beverages, have a snack, and play chess, or backgammon, or cards. Where people would hang out. Staple products would be antiques, maps, wall décor, smoking accessories and interesting imports from around the world. New and used books on the subjects of religion, geography, history, and art would support rotating displays on any topic that stuck. Great effort would be made to cater to people's interests. Also, effort would be made to introduce people to new things and Create interest.

The best part would be acquiring these marvelous products with travel to all points on the globe. My software experience will be invaluable in setting up a thriving business and tracking the large amount of data. This could also blossom into a restaurant where my experience is great.

Tim's Business Logo's

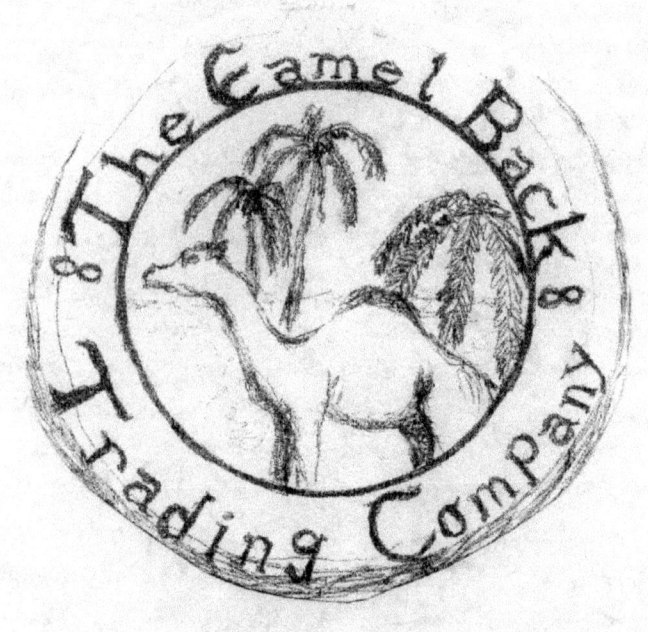

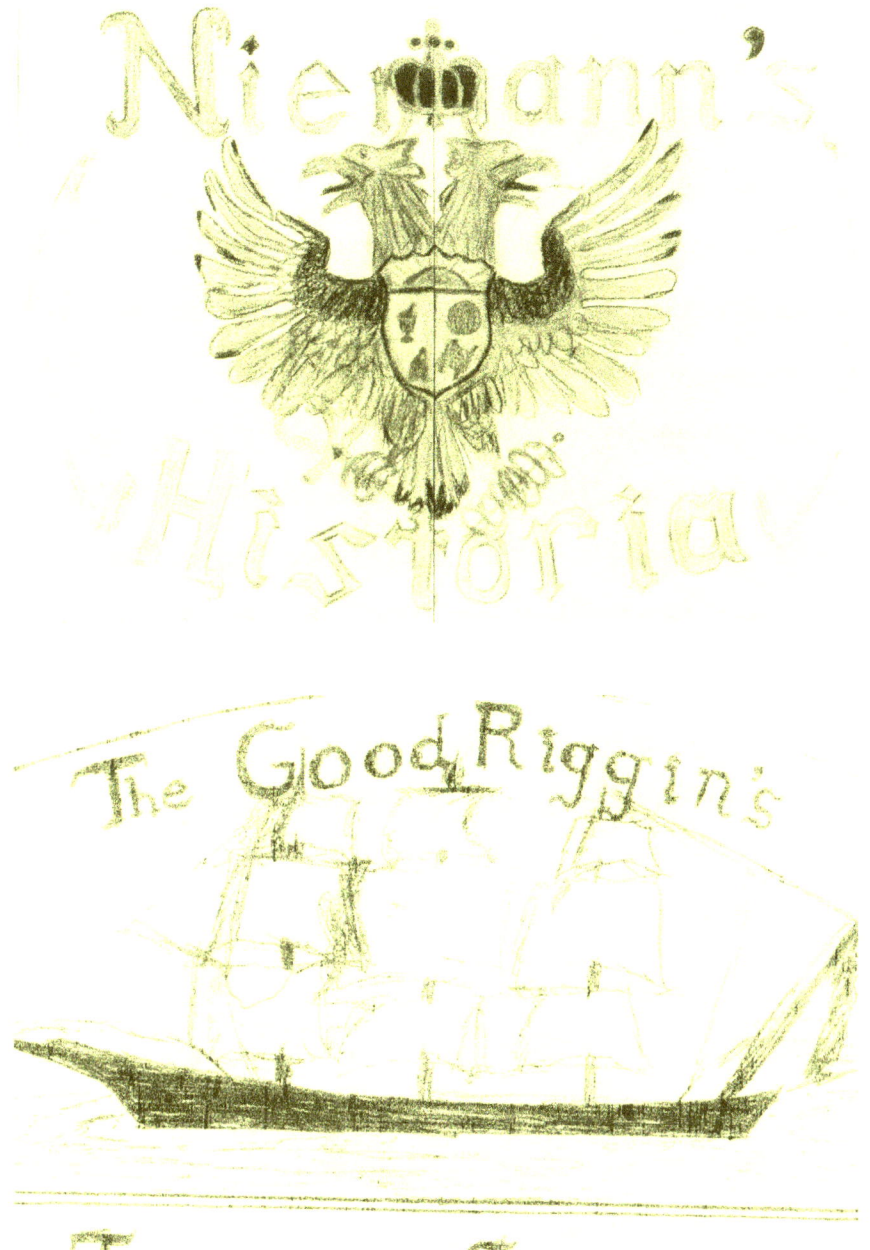

11

Tim's Poetry And Art

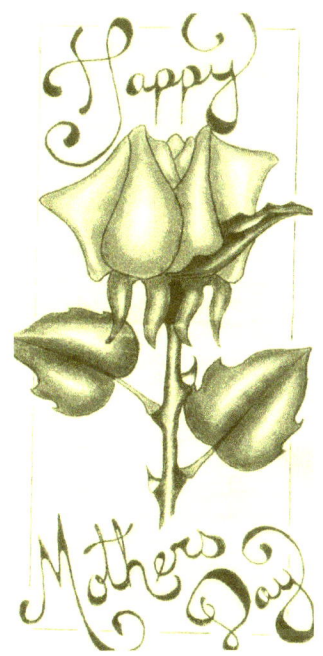

My Mothers Day Card

The inside of my Mother's Day card

SIMPLY BEAUTIFUL

My Mother loves the simple things,

The joy in a giggling child's eyes.

The warmth of an old man's smile.

Riches are not found with the King's,

But in doing what you are supposed to.

And with spreading a little love all the while.

Kindness is what my Mother brings,

Especially to those forgotten.

A caring smile at all life's trials,

My Mother has taught me many things,

Her walk in faith the most important,

Has made me feel worthy, and her simply

Beautiful.

Love,

Tim

BEST FRIENDS

While I'm forced to be away,

I think of you every single day

Not a moment goes by,

Without a silent cry,

Till I think of the time when we will play.

Best friends are never really apart,

Because the love between us shoots a dart.

That carries me with you

In everything that you do

And I thank God for the joy you impart.

Tim wrote this to Jennifer, his niece, in 1996.

Jennifer was eight years old

THANKS MOM

For

...always loving me

...being a great example

...providing a loving, stable, secure home.

...encouraging me

...helping me

...knowing how to have fun

...introducing me to God

...discipline

...loving everyone

...telling me I am capable

...being a Beautiful Person

I Love You,

Tim

Tim wrote this to me during his last year of high school.

Paul's Father's Day Card

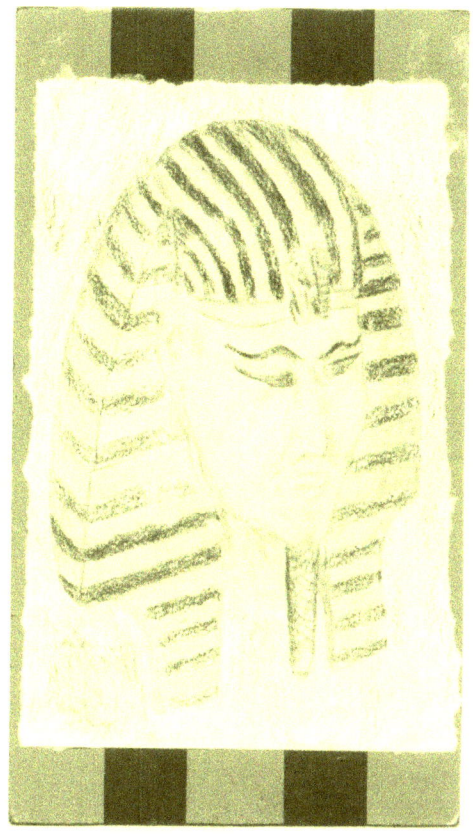

Paul's Fathers Day Card
The inside of Paul's card

HAPPY FATHER'S DAY

(June 15, 2001)

My Heart, my soul, everything I am,

Is the product of a special man.

No one can know what he means to me,

Because of his guidance, I am free.

From the time I lived as a child,
Maturing , but occasionally wild,
He allowed me the time, so I could see,
The kind of man that I could be.

Although I traveled a different path,
He wisely withheld his wrath,
So I would be able to know and believe,
Integrity like his is rarely achieved.

I am proud to be your son.

Love,
Tim

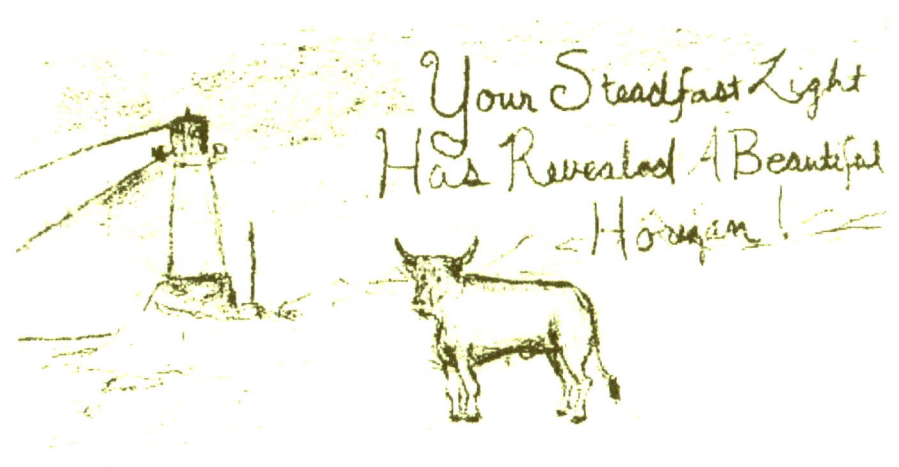

Your Steadfast Light Has Revealed A Beautiful Horizon!

HAPPY MOTHER'S DAY!

It takes a lot of Love

To Guide a Bull !!

I Love You.

Love Tim

Tim was born May 8, under the astrological sign of Taurus the Bull

99

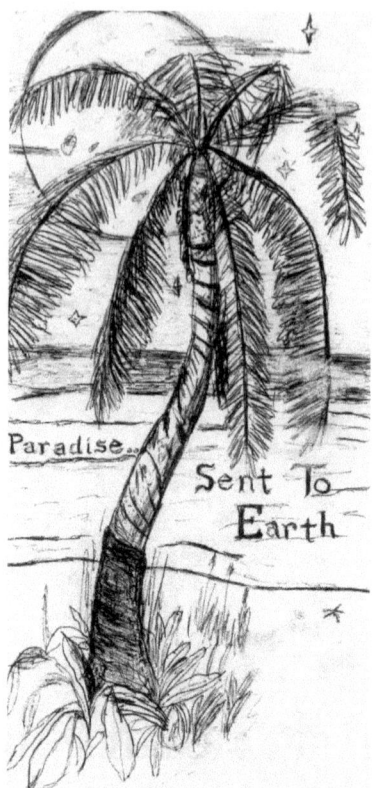

Merry Christmas

A special thanks for
your love and support,
A family like ours is
the finest present
one could hope for.

Love,

Tim

The following two poems were found in his files. They were typed and we are not sure if they are his words or not. They do sound like something he might write.

My soul a grey shadow is,

And tho with happiness I sometimes play

It seeks dark places

And shuns the light of joyous day.

It must be coaxed to dwell

Where crimson light is found

For in the secret of a shady dell

It dreams in soft sweet sound.

But like a ray of moonbeam

Or a fairy gleam of white

You steal into the shadow

And fill my soul with light.

Joy in the rain drop

Joy in the sun's rosy gleam

Joy that fills the spirit

With a never ending dream.

Birds afar off singing

Flowers opening bright blue eyes

Dancing in the woodland
Underneath the glorious skies.

Joy of youth and song of sorrow
Form the long long way
Which only leads on higher
Where fairer fields may lay.

TIMOTHY'S THOUGHTS

What's so wrong? Hard work is an idyllic profession:

Games played without favoritism or violence,

Games played among like-minded people,

And with laughter;

And family forgiveness and love.

What so wrong believing in all that?

What happened to the good sense I had at nine, ten,

eleven years of age?

How have I come to be such an enemy and player of

my self?

And so alone!

Nothing but self, locked up in me!

Yes, I have to ask myself — what has become of my

purposes.

Home? I have none!

Family? No!

One of our daughters was so hurt when she read this. I told her that I took the words "no family" to mean that he wasn't married and had no children.

12

Papers from Tim's Files

List the 'plus' about you

Smart

Good Athlete

Get along well with others

Look good

Willing to try new things

Learn quickly

Care about people

List the 'minus' about you

Irresponsible

Selfish

Immature

Get very depressed

Don't take care of money

Don't take care of myself

Get aggravated when people don't pay attention to me

Impatient

Are You Ready to List Some of Your Goals?

Lifetime – Have a family and learn to live responsibly

5 Years – Live out West or on the Ocean Coast

1 Year –   Be secure in my job and finances

Immediate – Learn to accept and take care of my illness

Another Page of Goals

Travel, where ever

Get to Germany

Finish degree

Find a technical job

Make a lot of money – $50,000 year and up

Quit smoking

Get in shape

Stay out of trouble

Start a business

Learn more about computers, how to make games

Stay close to God

Play sports

Position where I am part of a team, hopefully a leader

Stick up for myself

Girlfriend

Go to law School

Overcome fear

Get out of jail

Start painting and job brokerage company with Russ

Become Senator

Look into upgrading old computers and selling them

Learn German

Proud Feelings

1. What is something you are proud of that you can do on your own?

Get a good job

2. What are you proud of in relation to your family?

That my nieces love to see me because I'm funny

3. What is something that you are proud of that you made with your own hands?

Baked Chicken

4. What is a funny thing that you did about which you are proud?

Sent an official e-mail to a co-worker stating that the net admin. had found a game on his work station

5. What is a habit that you worked to overcome and succeeded, and are proud of doing so?

To quit being irritated of everyone, patience

6. Can you think of a decision that you made that you feel proud about, which required considerable thought?

Admitting that I needed Psych help and substance abuse help.

7. Think of a task you completed that was very hard (laborious) that you feel proud about?

Framed a bunch of prints for my apartment.

8. Think of a way in which you helped your family that you feel proud about.

Fixed my Mother's couch after my niece pushed a cushion out of place.

9. Can you think of a new skill that you've learned in the past year and which makes you feel proud?

Learned to send informational e-mails at work to keep people aware of developments.

10. Can you think of a time when you spoke up and said something and it took courage; when it would have been easier to remain quiet?

Spoke to boss about on-call rotation to tell him that his plan was not very workable.

SUPPORT GROUP

1 = point   = never true

2 = points = seldom true

3 = points = often true

4 = points = always true

Put the number that best fits you in the blank beside each statement

__3__   1. I am afraid to let other people get close to me. (trying to protect myself)

__2__   2. I fear the unexpected.

__2__   3. I look for the flaws instead of the shine in most situations.

__3__   4. I feel unworthy of other people's love.

__2__   5. I feel inferior to other people.

__4__   6. I have a compulsive habit, such as overworking, over eating, gambling, compulsive shopping, or alcohol or drug addiction.

__2__   7. I neglect my own needs in favor of caring for the needs of others

__3__   8. I have a lot of buried feelings from the past, such as anger, fear, shame, or sadness.

__4__   9. I seek approval and affirmation from others through people-pleasing, perfectionism or compulsive over-achievement.

__3__ 10. I take myself too seriously and find it hard to be playful and have fun.

__2__ 11 I have developed health or physical problems from excessive worry, stress or burnout.

__3__   12.   I have an overpowering need to control.

__2__   13.   I have difficulty expressing my true feelings.

__2__   14.   I dislike myself.

__2__   15.   My life seems to be in crisis.

__1__   16.   I think that I am a victim of life

__1__   17.   I am afraid of being abandoned by those I love.

__1__   18.   I criticize myself or put myself down.

__1__   19.   I expect the worst out of most situations.

__3__   20.   When I make a mistake, I feel that I am the mistake.

__1__   21.   I blame others for the troubles that befall me.

__2__   22.   I live in the past.

__2__   23.   I am closed to new ideas or different ways of doing things.

__2__   24.   I spend a lot of time being upset or angry about things that happen to me.

__2__   25.   I feel lonely and isolated even when surrounded by people.

__55__   Total Score

Supportive Relationships

1. **What would a supportive person say to you?**

   You look great

2. **What would a supportive person do for you?**

   Take me to the doctor

3. **What would a supportive person do with you?**

   Go to a movie

4. **What does "private" mean to you?**

   Things I want to control who knows

5. **Why do people need to keep some thoughts to themselves sometimes.**

   Make others uncomfortable

6. **What happens to you if you tell everyone everything all the time?**

   They do not want to listen

7. **How does that affect the way people treat you?**

   Do not take you serious

8. **What type of information do you feel comfortable sharing?**

   Events of the day

9. **Who are you the most comfortable sharing private information with?**

   My sister

I AM SPECIAL

I am special in all the world, there is nobody like me.

Since the beginning of time there has never been another person like me. Nobody has my smile. Nobody has my eyes, my nose, my hair, my hands, my voice. I am special. No one can be found who has my handwriting. Nobody, anywhere, has my taste - for food or art. No one sees things just as I do.

In all of time there has never been anyone who laughs like me, no one who cries like me. And what makes me laugh and cry will never provoke identical laughter and tears from anyone else, - ever. No one reacts to any situation just as I react. I am special!

I'm the only one in all of creation who has my set of abilities. Oh, there will always be somebody who is better at one of the things I'm good at, but no one in the universe can reach my quality or combination of talents, ideas, abilities, and feelings. Like a room full of musical instruments, some may excel alone. But none can match the symphonic sound when all are played together. I am a symphony.

Through all of eternity no one will ever look, talk, walk, think, or do like me. I am special. I am rare. And, as in all rarity, there is great value. Because of my great rare value, I need not attempt to imitate others. I will accept - yes, celebrate - my differences.

I am special! And I'm beginning to realize it's no accident that I am special. I am beginning to see that God made me special for a very special purpose. He must have a job for me that no one else can do as well as I can. Out of all the billion's of applicants, only one is qualified, only one has what it takes.

That one is me. Because …I am special.

"The Weaver"

"My life is but a weaving
Between my God and me,
I may not choose the colors
He knows what they should be.

For he can view the pattern
Upon the upper side,
While I can see it only
On this the underside.

Sometimes he weaveth sorrow
Which seemeth strange to me,
But, I will trust His judgment
And weave on faithfully.

'tis he who fills the shuttle
He knows just what is best
So I shall weave in earnest
And leave with Him the rest.

At last, when life is ended,
With Him I shall abide
Then I may view the pattern
Upon the upper side.

Then I shall know the reason

Why pain and joy entwined

Was woven in the fabric,

Of life that God designed."

Author: Benjamin M. Franklin

In Tim's files, we found a paper that had the words and music to the hymn 'Grace Greater Than Our Sin'. Tim and I talked many times about how God can forgive our sins. It was very important to Tim, but he couldn't see how God could forgive him.

Grace Greater Than our Sin

Marvelous grace of our loving Lord,

Grace that exceeds our sin and our quilt,

Yonder on Calvary's mount out-poured,

There where the blood of the Lamb was spilt.

Sin and despair, like the sea waves cold,

Threaten the soul with infinite loss.

Grace that is greater, yes, grace untold,

Points to the refuge, the mighty Cross.

Dark is the stain that we cannot hide.

What can avail to wash it away?

Look! There is flowing a crimson tide;

Whiter than snow you may be today.

Marvelous, infinite, matchless grace,

Freely bestowed on all who believe!

You that are longing to see His face,

Will you this moment His grace receive?

REFRAIN

Grace, grace, God's grace,

Grace that will pardon and cleanse with-in!

Grace, grace, God's grace,

Grace that is greater than all our sins!

Text: Julia H. Johnston

In one of the rehabilitation facilities Tim attended, a woman gave him a copy of 'Desiderata'. He liked it very much.

Desiderata

Go placidly amidst the noise and the haste, and remember what peace there may be in silence. As far as possible without surrender be on good terms with all persons. Speak your truth quietly & clearly; and listen to others, even to the dull and the ignorant; they too have their story.

Avoid loud & aggressive persons, they are vexations to the spirit. If you compare yourself with others, you may become vain or bitter; for always there will be greater and lesser persons than yourself.

Enjoy your achievements as well as your plans. Keep interested in your own career, however humble; it is a real possession in the changing fortunes of time.

Exercise caution in your business affairs; for the world is full of trickery. But let this not blind you to what virtue there is; many persons strive for high ideas; and everywhere life is full of heroism.

Be yourself. Especially, do not feign affection. Neither be cynical about love; for in the face of all aridity and disenchantment it is as perennial as the grass.

Take kindly the counsel of the years, gracefully surrendering the things of youth.

Nurture strength of spirit to shield you in sudden misfortune. But do not distress yourself with dark imaginings. Many fears are born of fatigue and loneliness.

Beyond a wholesome discipline, be gentle with yourself. You are a Child of the universe, no less than the trees and the stars; you have a right to be here.

And whether or not it is clear to you, no doubt the universe is unfolding as it should. Therefore be at peace with God, whatever you conceive Him to be, and whatever your labors and aspirations, in the noisy confusion of life keep peace with your soul. With all its sham, drudgery and broken dreams, it is still a beautiful world. Be cheerful.

Strive to be happy Max Ehrmann

Pages of Quotes That Tim Copied

Right Thinking

"We are all ready to be savage in some cause. The difference between a good man and a bad one is the choice of the cause."

-- William James

"To know that we have been eternally accepted by God in spite of all He sees in us and knows about us, is the root and ground of abundant life. God's acceptance is the secret to self-acceptance, and the seeking acceptance in the sight of men. We are filled with confidence, our guilt is gone, our conscience purged, our fears cast out; perhaps alone, but never lonely, we are made well by the miracle of His love".

-- H.L. Roush Sr.

"Jesus said her great love was due to her sense of having been forgiven much. The much that you have been forgiven will be unfolded a day at a time in your heart."

-- H. L. Roush Sr.

"The way to change others' minds is with affection, not anger."

-- The Dalai Lama

"The Transformed Mind"

"Fight the tendency to quit while you're behind."

-- Dave Weinbaum

"Whatever you want to do, do it now. There are only so many tomorrows."

-- Michael Landon

"You'll never be happy if you can't figure out that loving people is all there is - and that it's more important to love than to be loved."

-- Gwyneth Paltrow

"The job of a citizen is to keep his mouth open."

-- Gunter Grass

"You can make the world so much larger simply by acknowledging everyone else's."

-- Jeanne Marie Laskas

"The only failure is not knowing how to be happy."

-- Celine Dion

"Decide what your priorities are and how much time you'll spend on them. If you don't, someone else will."

-- Harvey Mackay

"It takes a lot of courage to show your dreams to someone else."

-- Erma Bombeck

"Don't confuse having a career with having a life. They are not the same."

-- Hillary Rodham Clinton

"There was never a night or a problem that could defeat sunrise or hope."

-- Bern Williams

"A window of opportunity won't open itself."

-- Dave Weinbaum

"Doing the best at this moment puts you in the best place for the next moment."

-- Oprah Winfrey

"They always say time changes things, but you actually have to change them yourself."

-- Andy Warhol

Ideas Worth Remembering

"Life isn't meant to be easy, it's meant to be life. And no religion defended so tenaciously the ordinary dignity of living. Judaism stressed neither an after-life, an after punishment, nor heaven; what was worthy and good was here…We seek God so earnestly, not to find Him, but to discover ourselves.

Reflections of Lian Eliav, a character in "The Source", by James A. Michener

"Oh, Lord, lead me from the unreal to the real. Lead us from darkness into light."

-- Hindu prayer

"Three tips for deep and simple living, common to every great tradition: spiritual practice, simplicity, and a dedication to service."

-- unknown

"The one task given to every man is to live life as a spiritual journey - never to be forgotten."

-- unknown

Resent Someone

"The moment you start to resent a person, you become his slave. He controls your dreams, absorbs your digestion, robs you of your peace of mind and goodwill, and takes away the pleasure of your work. He ruins your religion and nullifies your prayers. You cannot take a vacation without his going along.

He destroys your freedom of mind and hounds you wherever you go. There is no way to escape the person you resent. He is with you when you are awake. He invades your privacy when you sleep. He is close beside you when you drive your car and when you are on the job. You can never have efficiency or happiness. He influences even the tone of your voice. He requires you to take medicine for indigestion, headaches and loss of energy. He even steals your last moment of consciousness before you go to sleep. So - if you want to be a slave-harbor your resentments!"

-- anonymous

I do hope this book gives you an insight to the thinking and feelings of a person suffering with a mental disorder as my son, Tim, did for many years.

Susan's Thoughts of Tim

I saw a homeless man on the way home from my brother's funeral. For the last several years, when I would see someone begging on the entrance or exit ramp, I would think, that would be Tim if not for my parents. I would have, probably, more sympathy than most and would wonder what would happen to Tim after my parents were gone and my sister and I were in control of his demise. That tortured me. I loved my brother and had some great memories of him, but did not know if I was willing to turn my families life upside down to keep him from being one of those homeless people, begging on the ramps. I looked at this man with more compassion than I normally would have. I wondered, if he at some time in his life, had the support my brother had. I wondered if his family had given up on him years ago. What was different this time, looking at this homeless person, I wondered what his family had been through. My family had clearly been through hell.

Tim's life should have been an easy one. He was very intelligent, valedictorian of his graduating class. Excelled in most any sport he cared to pursue and made friends quite easily. Growing up we moved a few times. This was always a traumatic experience for my sister and me, who were both a little on the shy side, but Tim seemed to always have friends and lots of them right away. Yet his life was anything but easy. I think he always felt that there was too much expectation on him. Everyone was sure he would do great things with his life. His life turned out to be anything but easy.

He went away to college after he graduated high school. He first went to Purdue University and then Ohio University. He even made the Deans list at O.U. But his partying and mental problems got in the way of him ever having a degree. I remember him telling me of reaching such a low point at O.U. that he had considered suicide. I was horrified, but at the same time didn't take it as serious as I probably should have. I don't even think I ever told my parents. I had promised not to, and thought he was over reacting to the stress of college life.

I don't remember when he got his first D.U.I., but I do know he was young. It started out with thinking, he just had a drinking problem and all would be alright if he could just stop. His life became a series of jail time and rehab. After either, it would seem he had "seen the light" then the demons would always come back. It seems like every time they came back they were stronger, more in control and more difficult for Tim to fight off. That was still the early days when jail time was D.U.I.'S and the rehab was alcohol related.

It was during this time that my daughter was born. Tim was 23 years old at the time. He loved kids and it was obvious very early in Jennifer's life that she adored him. My mother admitted to feeling jealous of Jennifer's attention towards Tim. When he was in the room, it seemed like no one else was there, to her. They would laugh and have fun in their own little world. She was a toddler when Tim had gotten into difficulties with my parents and they had told him he had to move out of their house. I let him move into our home. I gave him a few simple rules that could not be broken. They were all broken, plus some I had not had the insight to make, and very early into his stay. He then went to his best friend, Russ, one of the few people who always supported him and would not say no. It broke my heart to tell Tim to leave, but I had no choice.

He ended up in jail shortly after that with another D.U.I. I always struggled with what to tell Jennifer. She loved him so much and I didn't want my anger to influence her opinion of him. I took her to visit him and wondered the whole time if I was doing the right thing for her. I did eventually refuse to let her visit him in jail. I spoke no bad words about him and kept my anger to myself. She was still a toddler at the time and adored her Uncle Tim. It was years later before she felt the anger and the pain.

Jennifer turned six shortly after we moved to Alabama. Every summer she would spend at least a couple of weeks with my parents. When she was eight, and made the trip, she came home very quiet. It took weeks for her to tell me what was bothering her. Tim, finally had his own place, and Jennifer was very excited about it. Shortly after arriving in Toledo, Grandma and Jennifer went to see Tim. He eventually came out on the porch, not opening the front door. She never was allowed inside the house that she was so excited about. Several weeks after she came home, while we were riding in the car, she started describing Tim's house. She then went into detail of what happened and why she hadn't seen the inside of Tim's house, in fact, she never saw Tim the rest of that trip. That was the first time that she felt the true reality and pain of what it was like to love Tim.

Tim was eventually diagnosed as Bi-polar. It explained a lot, but I always struggled with how much do you forgive and blame on a mental disorder. You can't live your life doing whatever you want, no matter what the consequences, and blame it all on a mental disorder. You can't steal, use drugs and rake havoc on your families' life with no blame. There are drugs to treat these conditions, but we are relying on mentally ill people to take them like they should. It should be of no surprise to us that they most often decide that they don't need them anymore and quit taking them, only to go back to the demons taking over their lives. I asked Tim once why he quit taking his lithium. He explained that there were side affects that were not pleasant and he would start feeling so much better and in control on the medication, that would feel he didn't need it anymore. This was a very intelligent person. He knew when he was answering that question that it really didn't make sense to quit taking the drug that was helping him so much.

I loved my brother and miss him terribly. He was so much fun to be with when he was doing well, but I am relieved that my parents life has been made easier.

A Few Concluding Thoughts

As the mother of a bipolar son, I often felt so alone. When people did not understand what we were going through, I would try not to mention Tim. If your friends or family are dealing with someone with problems, such as mental disorders, please try to empathize and give them support. A daughter of a friend of mine, here in our community, was so glad that she could come to me and talk openly about her bipolar son. I could understand and give her comfort.

Researchers are still learning about bipolar disorder. When Tim lived in Colorado, he had an excellent Psychiatrist, seemed to know much more than most doctors about bipolar. The sad thing was that the company Tim was working for changed insurance companies and the doctor was no longer in their plan. But he asked Tim one day if there was a time of the year when he had the most trouble. Tim's answer was yes, the fall. The doctor said the air pressure change has a great deal to do with that. I have only heard one other person mention this. Tim was living with us in Florida when the hurricanes hit a few years ago, and he could feel a change in his moods.

One time, while we still lived in Ohio, Tim said to me, "Mom, you haven't had a good birthday for a long time have you?" My birthday is October 3. I had to admit I hadn't. The Fall after Tim's death, Paul took me to my favorite place for my birthday - Great Smoky Mountain National Park. We rented a log cabin in Townsend, Tennessee. I love driving through Cades Cove and seeing all the deer and the occasional bear. I enjoyed it, but it was really too soon after such a tragedy.

People who suffer with the bipolar disorder become addicted to any addictive substance they consume. Also, the drugs and alcohol cover up the feelings, which are caused by their disorder. They feel better drunk than sober, if they are having an episode. I was told by a doctor that when they stop taking their meds for a period of time, it usually takes a higher dose to level their mood again.

So many bipolar people seem to be so violent, but thank goodness, Tim never was to us. I have always tried to treat people who have mental problems, with compassion and talk to them with respect. They also frequently have problems holding jobs, so they don't have medical insurance. They can't get life insurance, because they have a higher risk of suicide. We tried to increase the life insurance we had purchased when Tim was born, but they wouldn't because of his illness.

Something that sticks in my mind is Tim always complained about the nurses in the jail system. They would bring the meds at a certain time and if the person wasn't up at the cell bars, they did not get their medication. A Bipolar person has periods of time that they cannot sleep and then times that they can't stay awake. Their medications are so important. I found in his files, inmate papers where Tim was begging for his medication, for he felt so horrible. All of his papers were filed so neatly, it really amazed me that he kept everything.

The hardest thing I had to do was to call the Sheriff's Agency when I knew it had to be Tim who stole the van. But I thought of the poor person who worked hard to have a vehicle and now he had none. Tim needed help and I didn't know what else to do. I had tried everything I knew.

Sheriff Judd allowed me to attend the Crisis Intervention class one week with nineteen of his deputies. It was very interesting, and I now know of places where people with mental issues can go for help. The agency is using Tim's journal and his other writings in its crisis intervention classes.

I would like to thank the deputies that I have come in contact with since we moved to Florida. They have all been so very kind to me and they did try to help Tim find the treatment. I applaud Sheriff Judd and his agency for what they are doing to help the mentally ill.

Timothy was embarrassed that he wasn't able to keep a job and own possessions like his old friends did. So many times, I think how sad it is when such a beautiful, creative person's life goes to waste because of illness, drugs, and alcohol. I wish I could have helped Tim succeed in life, but I think God had other plans.

I love you Timothy, and I miss you!

www.ingramcontent.com/pod-product-compliance
Lightning Source LLC
Chambersburg PA
CBHW051320170526
45166CB00002B/622